The Hellers have written a very practical and lucid guide to dealing with and, more importantly, healing from the trauma of an auto accident. As body therapists we work with the residual effects of traumatic events—pain, dysfunction, and emotional suffering—on a daily basis. We have found the information in this manual to be a very powerful tool in assisting our clients to fully resolve their trauma symptoms.

—Avadhan Larson, L.Ac., Upledger Certified Craniosacral Therapist
—Dick Larson, L.Ac., Certified Advanced Rolfer

This book has been an invaluable resource for treating trauma patients. My training as a therapist has been in talk therapy. We know now that this does not work. The Hellers' book and training has helped me tremendously in treating these patients. They write in clear, simple language which make it user friendly. Their stories and examples are extremely helpful and valuable as we work with people who have had automobile accidents and/or experienced trauma in their lives.

—Barbara M. Dalberg, Ph.D., L.P.C., Psychotherapist

Diane Heller helps us understand why traditional psychotherapies may be unsuccessful in treating clients with posttraumatic stress responses due to auto accidents. The simplicity of her therapeutic approach belies its profound impact.

—Lesley L.Evans, Ph.D., Psychotherapist Adjunct Faculty,
University of Colorado and University of Northern Colorado

Diane Heller shines her light on a neglected aspect of modern life, dealing with the consequences of auto accidents. I don't know anyone who won't be changed by this helpful and hopeful book. It contains amazing insights and practical suggestions for average folks and therapists alike. Highly recommended!

—Robert W. Blackburn, Ph.D., California State University, Hayward

The treatment of trauma is never an easy task. Here is a manual for auto accident victims that really works. The Hellers and their trainees are making a difference without retraumatizing their clients. Everyone who has experienced an auto accident and those practitioners who treat them can benefit from reading this book.

—Jim Jonell, Ph.D., CareerLab, Vice President of Operations

Having treated many victims of trauma particularly from car accidents, I recognize the necessity of addressing the nervous system factors related to trauma, as these factors may continue to affect mental, emotional, social, as well as physiological function. Diane and Larry provide an excellent and vital tool for assessing and addressing imbalances created by trauma that can make profound changes in those who suffer from the effects of a car accident.

—Russell Sher, D.C. Chiropractor

I wish that this information had been available twenty-five years ago when I had my first auto accident. Three auto accidents later, I was blessed to discover Diane Heller and her approach to recovery. This book offers hope and healing to anyone whose life has been altered by a traumatic auto accident.

—Peggy Dennis, CMT, Denver, Colorado

When you're a working mother, you drive. No choice—not driving is not an option. I was in the car easily ten hours per week and I was in agony. I could hardly breathe, my face was oddly numb, and I often visualized the steering wheel breaking off in my hands. Driving on the highway was out of the question. The road to recognizing my condition as panic attacks was ridiculously long (and I'm a doctor!). Fortunately, the path from there to Diane Heller's office was fortuitously short. Her remarkable therapeutic technique transported me mentally back to the previous year's auto accident that had set off all this bodily chaos, then brought me back in a kinder, gentler way, nearly free of the terror. . .and all this in the first one hour session. As I hopped on the highway on my way home from her office that day, my breathing was free and easy for the first time in months. I am grateful to be free of that suffocating physical fear.

—Judith Paley, M.D., Capital Hill Internal Medicine, Denver, Colorado

Believing in the resilience of the human spirit, and knowing how to restore a person's confidence to use that ability for the recovery from trauma, is Dr. Heller's wonderfully effective approach to healing trauma.

—Dr. Cynthia Lawrence-Wallace, Professor Emeritus, University of California San Diego, Faculty of Western Institute for Social Research, Berkeley, California

In this book Dr. Heller provides tangible suggestions, realistic hope and support, and a conceptual framework for people who are recovering from the trauma of auto accidents. The ideas and suggestions put forth are concrete, as well as intellectually solid. Of special significance is "The Heller Resiliency Scan" which gives step by step guidance in how each person can identify the resources in his or her life that can aid their healing process. This is an invaluable aid to self-help efforts for those recovering from all types of trauma and indeed, the book should be quite helpful to survivors of various kinds of trauma, as well as to the professionals who treat and assist trauma survivors. Diane's emphasis is on "what's right with people" and how we can use this knowledge to heal ourselves and assist others in healing. This book is unique in the way it interweaves insight from years of clinical practice with further scholarly research and then translates all this into concrete, useable knowledge and wisdom. I will be recommending this book to students, fellow academicians and friends for years to come.

—John Bilorusky, Ph.D., President, Western Institute for Social Research, Berkeley, California

Diane Heller has done a superb job helping car accident victims understand and recognize the bewildering effect that their traumatic experience has on them; more importantly she helps them heal themselves through very clear and effective exercises. She has brilliantly been able to translate to the public the theory and technique of Somatic Experiencing in simple lay terms while permitting a deep understanding of what's going on at the bodymind level after a trauma. While her book addresses car accident victims in particular, it can benefit victims of all kinds of trauma. It is very helpful for health practitioners as well.

—Gina Ross, MFCC, Los Angles, California

CRASH COURSE

A Self-Healing Guide to Auto Accident Trauma & Recovery

Diane Poole Heller, Ph.D.
With Laurence S. Heller, Ph.D.

Foreword by DR. PETER A. LEVINE
Author of *Waking the Tiger*

North Atlantic Books
Berkeley, California

Crash Course: A Self-Healing Guide to Auto Accident & Recovery

Published by North Atlantic Books
P.O. Box 12327
Berkeley, California 94712

Printed in the United States of America

Cover and book design by Jan Camp

Crash Course is sponsored by the Society for the Study of Native Arts and Sciences, a nonprofit educational corporation whose goals are to develop an educational and crosscultural perspective linking various scientific, social, and artistic fields; to nurture a holistic view of arts, sciences, humanities, and healing; and to publish and distribute literature on the relationship of mind, body, and nature.

North Atlantic Books' publications are available through most bookstores. For further information, call 800-337-2665 or visit our website at www.northatlanticbooks.com.

Substantial discounts on bulk quantities are available to corporations, professional associations, and other organizations. For details and discount information, contact our special sales department.

Library of Congress Cataloging-in-Publication Data
Heller, Diane
   Crash Course: A Self-Healing Guide to Auto Accident Trauma & Recovery / by Diane Poole Heller with Laurence Heller.
       p. cm
   ISBN 1-55643-372-7 (alk. paper)
   1. Traffic accidents—Psychological aspects. 2. Post-traumatic stress disorder—Treatment. 3. Traffic accident victims—Rehabilitation. 4. Self-care, Health.
   I. Heller, Laurence, 1944–. II. Title.
   RC552.P67 H445 2001
   617.1'028—dc21   2001030890
                                                                 CIP

      1   2   3   4   5   6   7   8   9 / 06   05   04   03   02   01

Contents

Contents

Contents

Acknowledgements

Although this book is written in my voice as Diane Poole Heller and is comprised of material I originally developed based largely on Dr. Peter Levine's Somatic Experiencing model for trauma recovery, my husband and professional partner, Laurence Heller, Ph.D., has been a part of this project from beginning to end. He wrote several sections of the book. He helped me organize and communicate those perspectives and provided clinical examples from his private practice.

Additionally, the work and assistance of others have influenced my career as a psychotherapist and trauma specialist. I would especially like to thank Peter Levine, Ph.D., founder of the Foundation for Human Enrichment (F.H.E.), for his groundbreaking work on the resolution of trauma. Peter developed the model called Somatic Experiencing and has dedicated his career to the scientific study of how to help human beings move through and renegotiate overwhelming life events without feeling overwhelmed in the process. His unique understanding that trauma is in the nervous system, not in the event; that symptoms are generalized and biologically predictable will be delineated at length in this book.

Peter helped found the F.H.E. to promote the healing of trauma. Larry and I both are on the faculty of this organization teaching these principles in the United States, Europe and the Middle East. The Foundation now sends teachers to these locations as well as to South America, Japan, Australia, and other countries around the world, training many thousands of practitioners in the principles and techniques of Somatic Experiencing.

Special gratitude goes to our staff and to those clients and seminar participants who have shared their experiences in their earnest journey toward transformation. They exhibit notable courage in risk-taking, and a willingness to stretch beyond the known into initially awkward new territories. Their willingness, openness and professionalism have enhanced our learning as well as their own.

With the deepest appreciation we want to acknowledge Carole Williams for her tireless efforts in assisting in the writing and organizing of this book. We also send particular thanks to Kevin Heller, Nelly Frisch, Tavia Campbell, Lynda Parker, and Nina O'Kelley for their excellent editorial contributions. Dr. Jim Jonell also did a fine job sharing his wisdom on teenage driving.

Foreword

Every year millions of people suffer bewildering symptoms in the aftermath of even minor automobile accidents. This book will not only help people and their doctors understand these symptoms, but will empower them with simple but powerful tools that can support in healing.

After an event such as an accident, we are automatically put into state of shock. This state is normal and is meant to protect us from physical and emotional pain. Normally this altered state of consciousness is supposed to dissipate after a short period of time. Unfortunately, however, this does not always happen.

When people do not complete what is normally a time limited reaction, they are likely to develop both physical and psychological symptoms. These are frequently confusing and frightening. Often when they seek help from health care professionals their helpers are also confused and frustrated. These elusive symptoms crawl all over the body like the Lilliputians in Jonathan Swift's classic novel, *Gulliver's Travels*. These symptoms invade the psyche as well. The physician or therapist, in frustration, may then conclude that their patients are "malingerers" or have some other vague "psychosomatic" or "hysterical" condition. This can make the individual feel more helpless, even desperate. In addition, this sad situation is frequently compounded further when litigation and insurance settlements are involved. These suffering persons may go from doctor to doctor with the same question. What is wrong with me? Is it something physical, or is it just in my head?

In this carefully thought out book, the Hellers show, through clear explanations and many case examples, that the symptoms these people experience not only are real, but can be understood, prevented, and healed. Because trauma resides in the body, as well as the mind, an approach that does not deal with mind and body together will have only limited success. The Hellers show that trauma is neither a physical nor a psychological problem. It is rather a problem of learning a normal response to an abnormal situation.

Drawing from Somatic Experiencing, a mind/body approach to the healing of trauma, the Hellers carefully inform and guide the reader in this healing journey. In doing so they help guide the reader in recovery, and at the same time, in the discovery of a deeper, more resilient, and powerful self.

Somatic Experiencing shows that trauma is not in the event but rather in the deregulation of the nervous system. It is for this reason that different people react to what appears to be the "same" event very differently. Hopefully, this knowledge will reduce the sting of self-blame that people have when they can not get over their symptoms.

When we experience a perceived threat, our nervous system is instantly aroused to mobilize us for survival. The energy involved for life-preserving defense is vast; it is the energy that allows a hundred pound mother to lift a car and rescue her trapped child even when her muscles tear and bones break. When we are sitting in our car, patiently waiting for the light to change and someone unexpectedly smashes into us from behind, that same kind of intense energy is mobilized, but in a fleeting moment. However, there is little that we can do to defend ourselves. We can not fight or flee, and unlike the heroic mother, there is no effective action for us to carry out. In that fraction of a second when our bodies are unexpectedly jarred, we can not respond purposefully. It is for that reason that the vast survival energy gets locked in our bodies and in our minds. It is as though it (the energy) is all dressed up with no where to go.

But that energy must go somewhere; and into the symptoms of trauma it goes. Our necks and backs brace and seize up in painful spasms. Our nervous system is so aroused that we cannot sleep or rest well. Our minds begin to fret in anxious worry. We may begin to develop a phobia of driving or more general anxieties. When this goes on for months we become fatigued and depressed from the pain, lack of sleep, and feelings of anxiety and helplessness.

This book offers reassuring assistance with the proverbial "ounce of prevention." The information and guided exercises can help prevent these symptoms from developing in the wake of automobile accidents that the majority of us will experience some time in our lives. It is a book that can help ease unnecessary suffering; it should come along with every operator's manual for your automobile or AAA membership. It is at least as valuable.

—Peter A. Levine, Ph.D.
Director of the Foundation Human Enrichment
Author of *Waking the Tiger: Healing Trauma*

How To Use This Book

This book is intended as a workbook to restore you to health and to help you regain a sense of well-being after an auto accident. The techniques you will be learning here are specifically designed to work with resolving trauma by breaking the experience down into one manageable piece at a time.

Feel free to proceed through the chapters at your own pace. You may find your attention span is shorter than it was before your accident. It is actually important not to go too quickly through the book. We will be referencing material that will reconnect you to your accident experience in a way that is specifically designed not to overwhelm you.

Examples in this Book

The examples throughout this book are drawn from clinical experience that my partner, Larry, and I have gained over the past several years specializing in treating clients with auto accident injuries and post-traumatic stress disorder or (PTSD). We have changed the names and details of the cases to protect the privacy of our clients but the essence of the situation is maintained. One or more of these cases may be similar to your own experience.

Throughout the book, you will be given exercises. These are examples of techniques used in our private practice and within the context of my workshops for many years. Many are based on Peter Levine's Somatic Experiencing Model. When you do the exercises, choose a quiet location where you feel safe. Sit in a comfortable chair. Do the exercises when you have time to concentrate and are not rushed.

Sometimes you may feel that you are living more in the time of the traumatic event than in the present, even if the overwhelming event occurred several years ago. I want to help you catch up to yourself and develop the capacity to live your life now with a sense of well-being, with less and less focus on trauma. Of course we can't change history but we've found that we can greatly reduce *how* trauma affects you in the present and in the future. Using these techniques, symptoms are often greatly reduced or alleviated without the use of drugs or lengthy therapy.

Through the material presented in to you this book, you will understand:

- Why low-impact fender benders can cause such severe symptoms

- Why it is important to work through the events of the accident non-sequentially

- How to evaluate the events surrounding the accident and how they affected you

- How to enhance your sense of resiliency and well-being while releasing excess energy trapped in your body from unresolved shock or freezing

- Why this treatment is often effective in a short time and how you can participate in your own healing

- How to restore your normal defensive responses, which are necessary for safe driving

- How to fill in your loss of memory regarding certain aspect of the accident

- How to overcome the shock of a high-impact collision to your nervous system

- How to understand the profound impact of ruptured boundaries and learning to repair them

- How to gently release whiplash and compression symptoms

- How to resolve a feeling of being trapped when you buckle your seat belt

- Why airbag impact can add to your trauma

- How to deal with the special problems of teenage drivers

- How to overcome feelings of guilt or grief if you were involved in an accident where someone died

- How to move beyond the experience of your accident feeling healed and more able to cope with everyday stresses.

We believe this book can be a significant support to auto accident victims and their families as well as the professional caregivers that treat them. Nevertheless it is a self-help book and as such has built-in limitations. You may need to seek professional help if you have not already done so.

Overview of Somatic Experiencing

Somatic Experiencing (SE) is a short-term naturalistic approach to the resolution and healing of trauma developed by Dr. Peter A. Levine. It is based upon the observation that wild prey animals, though threatened routinely, are rarely traumatized. Animals in the wild utilize innate mechanisms to regulate and discharge the high levels of energy arousal associated with defensive survival behaviors. These mechanisms provide animals with a built-in immunity to trauma that enables them to return to normal in the aftermath of a highly charged life-threatening experience.

Although humans are born with virtually the same regulatory mechanisms as animals, the function of these instinctive systems is often over-ridden or inhibited by, among other things, the "rational" portion of the brain. This restraint prevents the complete discharge of survival energies, and does not allow the nervous system to regain its equilibrium. The energy that is not discharged remains in the body, and the nervous system gets stuck in "survival mode." The various symptoms of trauma result from the body's attempt to manage and contain this unused energy.

SE employs the awareness of body sensation to help people renegotiate and heal their traumas rather than relive them. With appropriate guidance into the body's instinctive "felt sense," individuals are able to access their own built-in immunity to trauma, allowing the highly aroused survival energies to be safely and gradually discharged. When these energies are discharged, people frequently experience a dramatic reduction in or disappearance of their traumatic symptoms.

Because traumatic events are often encounters with death, they evoke extraordinary responses. The transformation process can allow people to deepen their sense of self and others. The healing journey can be an "awakening" of untapped resources and feelings of empowerment. With the help of these new capacities, people can open portals to rebirth and achieve an increased sense of flow. The experience can be a genuine spiritual awakening, one that allows people to reconnect to the world.

The very structure of trauma, including hyperarousal, dissociation, and freezing, is based on the evolution of predator versus prey survival behaviors. The symptoms of trauma are the result of a highly activated, incomplete biological response to threat, frozen in time. By enabling this frozen response to thaw, then complete itself, trauma can be healed.

Traumatic symptoms are not caused by the dangerous event itself. They arise when residual energy from the event is not discharged from the body. This energy remains trapped in the nervous system where it can wreck havoc on our bodies and minds. Wild animals have developed the ability to shake off this excess energy. The key for humans in dispelling traumatic symptoms lies in our ability to slowly activate and then discharge this excess energy as well. Somatic Experiencing provides very precise techniques to help a person do this.

—Peter A. Levine

Key Phrases

Because the techniques in this book are new to you, let's start by defining some of the key phrases.

ACTIVATION—Hyperarousal or overcharge of the nervous system.

AROUSAL—Charge in the nervous system

AUTONOMIC NERVOUS SYSTEM—The part of the nervous system responsible for involuntary functioning such as breathing, heart rate, perspiration, appetite, trembling, sleep, shaking, and sex drive, etc.

BOUNDARIES—The sense of personal space and containment that allows you to feel safe.

BOUNDARY RUPTURE—A feeling that you are no longer protected or sheltered from events and objects around you, of being flooded by outside stimuli.

CREATIVE SELF-REGULATION—The body's capacity to modulate activation and remain balanced. Modulation of activation means that the body has the energy it needs to face challenges or danger as well as the capacity to discharge and rest after a challenge has been met.

DISCHARGE—Release of energy through the body.

DISSOCIATION—Disconnection, "zoned" or "spaced" out.

FREEZE FRAME—The technique in which you capture a dangerous moment by stopping or "freezing" it like a frame in a movie. This use of stopping the image or action gives the body time to contact and complete its normal biological defense mechanism of fight or flight.

LINKING—The snapshot the mind takes of a traumatic event that then causes us to associate any element in that "snapshot" with danger, i.e, if we were hit by a white car on a highway in the mountains when it was raining, we may associate all of these elements (white cars, driving in the mountains, driving on highways, rainstorms) with threat afterwards which may trigger anxiety reactions.

LOOPING (PENDULATION)—The technique of moving from a resource, which promotes relaxation and discharge, to the experience of a small piece of traumatic material that is still upsetting. Then back and forth in order to make the process of trauma resolution less painful and more manageable.

NONSEQUENTIAL—Not in the order the event originally took place.

OASIS—An inner experience of safety that a person can rely on for support that is needed when beginning to work on difficult trauma material. You never work with the traumatic experience without first establishing this stable foundation called an oasis.

OVERACTIVATION—Overarousal and overcharge in the nervous system.

OVERWHELM—A state of feeling there is more than you can cope with at any given moment.

RANGE OF RESILIENCY—That range within a person based on genetics, family history, support system, etc., that allows a person to deal with life's difficulties without being overwhelmed.

REPTILIAN BRAIN—Core brain often referred to as "primitive" because it is the oldest part of our brain. Expert in survival, self-preservation, and instincts.

RESILIENCY—The capacity to cope with life challenges and remain connected to yourself in an integrated way. The capacity to "bounce back" after difficulty.

RESOURCE—Anything that makes you feel safe and comfortable, helps discharge your tension or arousal, and triggers a relaxation response.

SURVIVAL MODE—The state of hyperarousal where you are continuously mobilized to meet threat.

TITRATION—A healing process where you deal with the trauma one small, manageable step at a time, piece by piece, bit by bit.

WORKING THE PERIPHERY—Begin with the least traumatic material and slowly move toward the more traumatic material.

1

⮑

What Happens To You

During and After
an Automobile Accident?

One of the most dangerous things you will probably do today is drive your own car.
—Diane Heller

Who Should Read This Book?

Are you one of the seven million Americans who was involved in an automobile accident last year? Has someone you know or love been injured in an accident?

I've been injured in a serious auto accident myself, and I personally understand a lot of what you might be going through. In fact, it changed the course of my psychotherapy career. As a result, I've dedicated my professional life to treating victims of auto accidents and survivors of other types of severe traumas.

This book is written for two groups of people, as well as for their families and caregivers. First, it is for those of you who know you have lasting symptoms from your automobile accident, symptoms for which you have not been able to find relief. The other group is those of you who have been in an accident, maybe even some years ago, and are not aware of having lasting ill effects. Perhaps your appetite or your sleeping patterns have changed, or you are having mood swings, depression, anxiety or even physical pain you can't find a reason for. As you read this book, you will see how these behavior and mood changes, which may not have surfaced until months after your accident, can be directly related to the trauma you suffered in the collision.

Auto Accidents—An Everyday Event

In contrast to other extreme life events, auto accidents are so common that we often mistakenly take them for granted as a part of everyday life. A *Dateline* television program estimated that an auto accident occurs every two seconds in the United States. In other countries such as Israel, for example, the incidence is two-and-a-half times higher. Yet accidents can cause far-reaching reactions in our bodies that disrupt our quality of life, leave us unable to work, cost thousands of dollars in treatment, and exact untold hours of chronic pain or suffering. Some of these symptoms are easily recognized as the result of the accident. Others are not so easily recognized, but may be no less debilitating.

According to the National Center for Statistics and Analysis there were over six million auto accidents and over three million people injured in 1999 in the United States alone. A study reported in the *American Journal of Psychiatry* (April, 1999) showed that most auto accident victims showed symptoms of Post Traumatic Stress Disorder, that symptoms remain high more than nine months after the accident, and that women are more likely than men to suffer lingering symptoms. Histories of trauma or depression also increase the risk of lasting trauma, according to the study. Of course, not everyone who is in an auto accident suffers from Post Traumatic Stress. Post traumatic stress reactions will vary depending on the intensity of the traumatic event, previous trauma, your support system available after the traumatic event, your psychological history and genetic resiliency.

Could Your Symptoms Be Accident Related?

According to a paper, "Victims of Traffic Accidents: Incidence and Prevention of Post-Traumatic Stress Disorder," (Brom, Kleber and Hofman) accident victims tend to compulsively re-experience parts of the accident or the whole event. They have a tendency not to remember what has happened, be unwilling to discuss the event, or feel emotionally numb. They experience feelings of guilt, depression, behavioral changes, feelings of anger and anxiety, and sleeping disturbances that can last for months or even years.

"In most cases, traffic accidents involve a mixture of psychological, medical, and legal consequences that interact in a complex way," the paper states.

One group of accident victims we see in our practice consists of people who have had persistent moderate to severe symptoms since an auto accident—aches, pains, depression, and anxiety to name but a few. In this group we have many people who don't know that their symptoms relate to an earlier accident. Larry recently treated a woman for depression and anxiety that she thought was related to her marital situation. After five weeks of treatment, she recalled an accident that she had six years earlier. She had no idea it was still affecting her. After only two sessions of work on the accident her depression and anxiety were greatly reduced, giving her more energy to tackle her marital problems. In the course of those two sessions, she saw how a number of her symptoms were related. Why she had pain in her left shoulder, why she got so anxious when she was in the vicinity of her accident, and even why she started smoking again several months after the accident.

Here are some questions to ask yourself: Do you prefer to be the driver to feel more in control? Did you suffer whiplash in your accident? Have you felt anxious about driving ever since your accident? Do you wake at night suffering from nightmares or flashbacks about the accident? Do you still have pain or headaches that no amount of treatment seems to relieve? Do your anger and frustration seem to leak out everywhere? Do you avoid the spot where the accident took place? These are some obvious symptoms resulting from accidents.

Other symptoms include being more irritable than usual, gaining or losing weight, having trouble sleeping, finding yourself suffering from a lack of interest or a greatly increased interest in sex, or simply not feeling like yourself.

Strange as it seems, all of these symptoms can be direct results of your auto accident, even though they may not appear until up to 18 months later. It seems that our bodies are able to compensate for a while. When "mysterious" and/or persistent uncomfortable symptoms continue to show up, even months or years later, this book can help you understand possible causes and help you find relief from your symptoms.

Have well-meaning medical professionals suggested that your symptoms are all in your head? Do you fear you may be going crazy? Often when our symptoms become entrenched and our caregivers, no matter how well intentioned, are uncertain how to help us, we begin to blame ourselves. All too often when clients come to my office for an initial interview, they comment that they feel out of control of their lives and that they fear they are going crazy. This book is to help you understand why post-traumatic stress response may feel "crazy-making" but that you are not crazy! Given what happened to you, your trauma symptoms, if you have them, do make sense and often can be significantly reduced when understood and respected. The body is intelligent in its inherent wisdom regarding its own capacity to heal with the proper support. If I could build a billboard for trauma survivors it would say in bold letters, YOU ARE NOT CRAZY! Under that, I might add, YOU CAN HEAL! Your body knows how to heal.

This book can help you now by:

• Showing you that many of your symptoms are a normal result of trauma's impact on the nervous system.

• Offering case histories to illustrate that others have suffered similar symptoms and how they recovered.

• Providing exercises to be done alone, with a companion, or in conjunction with treatment from health professionals.

- Helping you learn how to relieve your symptoms in a safe and integrating way.

- Releasing survival energy trapped in your nervous system by the accident and making it available to you for other interests and activities.

- Teaching you resiliency-building techniques that will help you overcome past trauma and transform your life.

- Giving you skills that will greatly improve your way of meeting future challenges or dealing with trauma in the future.

The techniques in this book will change your life. Working with this book will give you a renewed sense of power and capability, a sense of "I can," and an awareness of new choices and abilities. Your fears related to driving and your symptoms connected to the accident should be greatly diminished or alleviated.

It Happened to Me

My own auto accident gave me a very personal interest in trauma therapy and methods for recovery. September 14th, 1988 is a day I will never forget. I was involved in a very serious high-velocity, head-on collision. And it occurred only two weeks before my greatly anticipated wedding day. Suffering a mild brain injury, (although at the time I didn't know what that was), I was left somewhat disoriented during, before, and after the big event. I was in a very confused state as I was scurrying to doctors' appointments in the midst of last minute floral and catering preparations. Still scared to death of driving, I was running around in an unfamiliar rental car because mine had been totaled. Not only did I have to buy a wedding dress, I had to negotiate on a new car when I couldn't even think straight. I couldn't remember how many people would be at the rehearsal dinner and gave the restaurant incorrect reservations because I couldn't add up the numbers. Everything that had been so organized began to crumble into chaos. The smallest decision became overwhelming and there were far too many decisions. Thankfully, Larry and I married on October 1 despite the difficult circumstances.

How did this head-on collision happen? Driving down a four lane undivided highway determined to finish up the final wedding details, I had my wedding organizer notebook on the seat beside me, along with a special porcelain ornament to decorate the top of our wedding cake. It was a beautiful porcelain bride and groom that had tremendous sentimental value. As an important symbol of my new family's tradition, this ornament had been used previously by my mother-in-law on her own wedding cake. She had given it to me as a gesture of generosity and as a warm welcome into the family.

What happened next was any future daughter-in-law's nightmare. As I was driving at 55 miles per hour, the wedding cake ornament began to slide on the slippery notebook cover. In a panic, I reached for the bride and groom, releasing my seat belt in order to catch the fragile piece before it smashed on the floor of the car. As the ornament slipped farther and farther toward the floor, I leaned over further and further. I got it! Yes! I had saved the bride and groom! I wasn't doomed as a first time daughter-in-law after all! Tradition was intact!

I looked up triumphantly only to see a Mercedes headed my way, filling my view and soon my windshield. In an instant I realized I'd twisted the steering wheel too far left, veering into oncoming traffic! It was too late. I was driving at a speed of 55 mph and so was the driver of the Mercedes. The combined impact was 110 miles an hour, and I did not have my seat belt on!

First I flew full force into the steering wheel, hitting my jaw above my front teeth. I cut the inside of my mouth and upper jaw. I also broke the windshield as the top of my head slammed into it.

I can recall at the same time, as if in slow motion, seeing the Mercedes I hit flipping in the air over my car, landing on the road upside down. I was certain the other driver must have been seriously injured or killed (thankfully, he wasn't). I was so concerned about him, of course, that I hardly noticed the miracle—that, although bloodied and banged up, I had survived.

The other driver not only survived, thanks to the substantial structure of his Mercedes, but he was uninjured and came to help me out of my crumpled car. He was an oral surgeon as well as a good Samaritan. He immediately was able to help with my facial injuries by giving useful instructions to the paramedics. From what I now know about trauma, I still wonder if he had symptoms that arose later. I have attempted to reach him since the accident, but I have not been able to find him to thank him or to find out how he is doing so many years later.

As a result of the accident and subsequent symptoms, I learned a great deal about what mild brain injury and high-impact accidents can do to people. I learned that when you are in high-impact shock it is a different dimension of injury. The experience may feel so fragmenting that you feel crazy and out of control inside. Your body gets deregulated, normal functions become "out of sync,"and previous traumas can be reactivated. For me it was like opening Pandora's box. Previous unresolved emotional issues resurfaced from the shock of the accident.

My delayed symptoms from the accident included strange temperature shifts from hot to cold and I experienced intense night sweats. I also awoke in the middle of the night with intense fear and intrusive flashbacks of the crash. I seemed destined to relive the event over and over again—as if once was not enough! It seemed I couldn't stop eating and I gained 30 pounds. I couldn't sleep past 3:00 a.m. I'd wake up feeling anxious. My whole body seemed out of whack.

One of the strangest symptoms I had for months afterwards was a compulsive need to act out the motions of buckling a seatbelt whenever and wherever I sat down! It made sense, though, when I thought about it. Because I had unbuckled my seatbelt just before the accident, moments before the life-threatening impact, the motions of undoing my seatbelt took on a special survival significance. From then on, anywhere I sat down, I automatically made the movement to buckle my seatbelt. This movement to buckle-up occurred at home, at the kitchen table, or while watching TV, at the office in my therapy chair, or even at the movies—an example of how trauma gets encoded in the body. I felt silly, but I couldn't stop myself from acting out the "buckle-up" scenario. I seemed to be trying to undo the damage over and over again. I was still stuck "in the accident" trying to save myself and attempting to prevent the crash. My life had been seriously threatened and all of my survival reactions had been mobilized. The problem was that they didn't turn off and were working overtime. I was stuck in survival mode.

Another interesting but potentially dangerous symptom became obvious to me only after a few loud honks from irritated drivers on the highway afterward. I somehow wasn't seeing traffic approaching on my left.

Merging onto highways became uncomfortable and difficult. Then I remembered more details about the crash.

At the instant of impact, I was twisted toward the left and was hit on the left side. I saw the oncoming car zooming toward me from the left just before impact. I desperately tried to steer the car to the right out of harms way—just not soon enough. Afterward, I found I couldn't look left without actually consciously forcing myself to move my head. In traffic I seemed to avoid looking left, which of course is an essential response for driving safely. I later learned my body was in "avoiding danger" mode, having identified the whole spatial relationship of left as "dangerous." I had in a sense "lost left." In other words, I had difficulty even being aware of cars, or anything else for that matter, coming toward me from the left. My reflexes and the capacity to orient in that direction, which we normally take for granted, were impaired. Survival for me then meant orienting to the right to get back to safety. It was as if I was still avoiding the oncoming Mercedes months after the accident was over!

I realized I was much more vulnerable to having another accident since I was not able to orient myself naturally in all directions. I began to feel a bit like a sitting duck in traffic. It was as if I could no longer trust my body's responses and instincts, a frightening realization indeed.

Talking about the accident increased my anxiety, even though that type of review was the treatment technique most people recommended. Although there were gaps in my memory, the parts I could remember, I couldn't stop remembering. I also began to experience the "Pandora's Box phenomenon" that I mentioned earlier. Unresolved traumas from the past and related symptoms were surfacing as powerfully as those from the auto accident. I had to find a way to deal with all of this fall-out. Traditional treatments weren't helping me much.

Because traditional medical and psychotherapy techniques weren't working well enough for me, my search for recovery possibilities took me nearly four years. I flew all over the country to a variety of trauma professionals seeking help before finding Peter Levine's Somatic Experiencing techniques. I subsequently used this technique as a basis for my own understanding. Thousands of people worldwide have been treated successfully using the Somatic Experiencing approach. I want to share this knowledge with you because I have found it so helpful for myself and many, many others.

Somatic Experiencing incorporates techniques and understanding from traditional medical, psychological, and physical therapies. What distinguishes Somatic Experiencing from these traditional treatments is how it identifies and works with what happens in the autonomic nervous system during an overwhelming life event. Therapists using techniques that emphasize retelling and reliving the event itself, including Critical Incident Intervention, can run the risk of unintentionally retraumatizing the people they are trying to help. As traditional practitioners integrate an understanding of how trauma affects the nervous system they find their own approaches are often greatly enhanced, thus more helpful to their patients.

Currently hundreds of medical and psychological professionals in over a dozen countries are being trained in Somatic Experiencing. Recently Larry and I trained a large group, including government officials, in Israel.

I learned that much of shock is experienced directly in the body, affecting us physically even more than emotionally or cognitively. I began personal treatment and extensive professional studies with Peter Levine. After a number of years and so many significant healing successes, I was impressed with the results and convinced that he really understood about how the body responds to traumatic stress, and more importantly, how to help reverse the process! Many scientists and researchers held the opinion at the time that once traumatized, a person's brain chemistry changed and could not be changed back. Drugs and coping skills for disabilities were often the only "cures" prescribed.

Eventually both Larry and I became teachers of Peter's work and faculty members of The Foundation of Human Enrichment, a non-profit organization dedicated to the healing of trauma founded in 1992.

Over subsequent years, I have developed a strong focus on empowerment, resiliency, and resourcing in my work with clients which I call The Heller Resiliency Model. I learned that moving through extreme trauma helps people call on powerful capacities within themselves; capacities that, as a hidden gift, can actually lead to a more stabilized existence than before they were injured.

As for the porcelain bride and groom figurine that caused the $60,000 accident, I did finally get it to the bakery in one piece. Ironically another incredible event took place that night. The little neighborhood bakery in Boulder had a break-in for the first time in its 15-year history. The bride

9

and groom statue, "safely" resting high up on a shelf atop the shop's CD player, was knocked to the floor and smashed to pieces when the burglars grabbed the valuable musical equipment. So much for my determined attempts to save it!

Why You May Not Know You Need This Book

Even minor fender-benders can trigger a response in your body that produces trauma. For many people who have been in accidents where there are no obvious injuries, symptoms such as insomnia, chronic pain, anxiety, and depression can seem totally unrelated to the event. Even medical practitioners may not be aware of the impact of minor accidents on the nervous system. This is partly because some symptoms don't surface clearly until days, weeks, or even months after the accident. As Somatic Experiencing treatment progresses it becomes more obvious how symptoms are related to the accident. Even though clients may believe their symptoms are totally unrelated, we know we are on the right track when, as we are working through the accident, we see their symptoms begin to lessen and resolve through the exercises and techniques we present here.

Read what happened to James, one of Larry's clients, who despite being a physical therapist and knowledgeable about trauma's effects on his clients, did not recognize his own accident's effect on him.

James

James was driving his MG at nearly 60 miles per hour when he lost control. His car hit the central barrier several times, banging him around inside the car. When the car stopped he was able to walk away from the accident. Paramedics verified that he had no obvious injuries despite sore muscles. James continued on to work as if nothing had happened. He didn't mention the accident to his boss or co-workers.

Not until weeks later did he realize he was not sleeping as well as before the accident. He felt edgy and irritable. Every time he drove near the location where he had his accident he became very anxious. Still, until he talked the problem over with Larry in a treatment session, he didn't identify his symptoms as possible results of the accident.

James's delayed reaction is common, as is his anxiety around the scene of the accident. You'll read in later chapters about your unconscious mind's ability to take in details of your surroundings at the moment of the accident. Afterward, your mind may associate these details, no matter how unrelated, to the actual danger of the accident itself. This explains why you may suddenly have a seemingly irrational fear of snow after the crash if it was snowing the day of the accident. Or you may feel fear when you see cars the same color as the one that hit you or even when you are in the part of town where your accident took place. You may feel extremely angry when a car approaches you too quickly from a certain direction. These types of triggers often happen when those details have become associated with the trauma of the accident.

Why We Need to Treat Auto Accident Trauma

Our lives revolve around automobiles. It is almost impossible to have a normal life in most areas of the United States without driving or riding in a car. The almost absolute necessity of having to continue to drive often triggers the original trauma. This book explains why auto accidents can change the way you orient to your surroundings, possibly making you more accident-prone in the future.

It's important for your safety and the safety of those on the road around you to resolve auto accident trauma. For instance, after a rear-end accident some victims may drive with almost all their attention focused on the rear-view mirror. Being so afraid of being hit from behind again makes them a hazard to themselves and to others on the road. After being previously rear-ended, one of my clients actually had another accident, running into a car ahead of her, because she was so intently watching the cars behind her.

It Isn't All In Your Head!

We live in a "get over it" culture. You may have found that your friends, family, or co-workers expect you to get on with your life and forget about the accident. Or you may be pretending that everything is fine because you think it is not normal to be so distressed weeks or months later. I want to reassure you that your reaction is perfectly normal. You may feel a little disorganized or crazy inside, you still may have strange pains, but *you are not crazy.*

Trauma is real. It can happen when the body's natural response to threat is interrupted or incomplete and if the level of feeling overwhelmed experienced exceeds the person's capacity to deal with it. You are not emotionally unstable or weak or crazy if you experience trauma symptoms immediately or even months after an accident. Your body is doing exactly what it was designed to do in an emergency. The trouble is, your body hasn't completed the cycle that nature intended. You're still in survival mode. The process of healing is thwarted. That's one of the reasons why you have symptoms.

This book explains what has happened to your body, how your nervous system gets overcharged, and how to complete the natural cycle and release the trapped energy that creates many of your trauma symptoms. When you face danger all your nervous system's energies of fight and flight are naturally mobilized. When you can't discharge this energy completely, what remains has to go somewhere—and can be expressed physically as headaches, stomach pain, or respiratory difficulties. Other times this unreleased energy will show up as emotional distress such as anger, anxiety, or phobia. Your ability to think clearly can be affected as well, leading to poor concentration or memory problems.

You may want to show this book to professionals with whom you are working so they can include the understanding of how trauma affects the autonomic nervous system with their approach to help you through the process of recovery.

What Makes This Approach Unique?

Your healing needn't involve a lifetime of therapy. Many of our clients need only 8 to 15 sessions to deal with auto accident trauma. Others require longer treatment. This book has been written with high hopes of helping you overcome your accident trauma as quickly and painlessly as possible.

You needn't spend months rehashing childhood issues like you do in some therapies. This book can help you work directly with your current symptoms and the specific events of the auto accident. We call it event-specific treatment. Working at home at your own pace, you should begin to obtain relief from your symptoms as soon as you have practiced a few of the simple exercises. Sometimes it is very helpful to have a partner that understands this way of working to help you.

Somatic Experiencing and my resiliency approach deal with biology, particularly the nervous system, to help you get back into balance. It explains what's happening in your body and that what you feel is a normal result of the trauma. After the accident, you may *feel* crazy or out of control, but you will begin to understand why your reactions are perfectly natural responses. This technique, like other therapies, deals with emotion and cognition. The emphasis, however, is on helping you re-regulate your nervous system and return to a sense of safety and well-being. In fact, use of the exercises and resiliency techniques in this book can give you a new, exciting outlook on life. Once the trauma is resolved, many clients feel their lives have been transformed in ways that affect all areas of their life. In addition, they often report that they are better, safer, and more skilled drivers than before the accident.

Why NOT To Tell People What Happened

Most therapies that deal with auto accident trauma encourage you to tell your story over and over again, start to finish, with the idea that talking about problems solves them. Somatic Experiencing works very differently. Whenever you tell the story your body is also listening and begins to respond to the sense of danger again and again. Repetition of the accident story can actually intensify the trauma, which overactivates the nervous system again. When the nervous system is overactivated you may feel flooded with stimuli, overwhelmed. You may lose focus and become unable to concentrate or remember things. If you become too overstimulated you may disconnect or "space out."

We emphasize helping you access and create physical and emotional resources for yourself to build a sense of resiliency. Enhanced resiliency can help you overcome traumatic events now and in the future. You will learn in this book that your own body has untapped resources that can help you regain wellness. Learning how to find and use your own inventory of personal resources can be an exciting journey. So often we get caught in focusing only on pain or what feels wrong in our bodies or our lives that we forget the invaluable awareness of what is working well. Usually when we are in physical pain, we lose contact with the parts of our physical self that still feel good. Often when clients come to us who have had chronic pain since their accident, they are surprised to find that there are areas in their body that still feel normal.

To heal we need to learn how to work with our pain and our symptoms as well as all of our natural resources. Using resources, explained in Chapter 6, helps your body relax and release trapped nervous system activation or excess energy, defusing the trauma. This allows you to come out of survival mode. Once your activation level is reduced and excess energy is discharged, you work through your accident non-sequentially. Remember, it's important not to tell the story of your accident in the order in which it occurred because you run the risk of reactivating the trauma in your physiology as happened in the accident originally.

David

One of Diane's clients, David Rippe, who requested that we use his real name and story in this book, had been in auto accident recovery treatment for several months. He suffered excruciating migraine headaches. With therapy he finally succeeded in reducing his headaches to a manageable level.

Then, despite Diane's concern, he gave a speech, retelling the events of his accident. Telling the story start to finish triggered a major headache episode and created a setback in his treatment. You will hear more about David's remarkable recovery in later chapters.

Instead of telling your story in sequence, it's preferable to start with your memories following the accident, especially focusing on when you first felt safe again. You may then touch in to memories from immediately before the accident when you first sensed something was wrong. You deal with the actual moment of impact, which is the most difficult, only at the end of treatment. Using exercises in this book, we will be teaching you how to switch back and forth between your "charged" experiences from the accident and the relaxing effect of your resources. This facilitates discharge and release in your nervous system.

Survival Is Success

One of the most obvious resources you can rely on at this point is that you *did* survive. Your body doesn't care how you survived the threat, whether you did it awkwardly or with great finesse. It just cares that you survived. Biological survival *is* success. Whatever you did worked. Now that you've survived, you have the opportunity to work through the residual injuries or symptoms from the experience you endured. When people get stuck in survival mode after an accident, it often is difficult for them to fully realize that they are now safe, that they have survived. They are so geared toward survival that they don't realize they've accomplished their goal. Part of them gets stuck in the event, which is one reason why they expect it to happen again.

> Reminder: If at any time you feel tired, stressed, or overwhelmed by what you are reading here, stop for a few minutes. When you feel able to continue, turn to the chapter on Resources and read it first. Reading about or discussing accident trauma can reactivate your original response to it.

Why Accidents Are So Traumatic

Some of the first reports of what we now call Post Traumatic Stress Disorder (PTSD) came after the invention of the railroad. Survivors of train crashes were treated for a condition called "railroad spine," known today as whiplash. Peter Levine prefers to call PTSD "post traumatic stress response," replacing disorder with response, because he believes that it is a natural physical response to an overwhelming event, not a disorder.

Even if your car is traveling at five miles per hour during a collision, it can cause a traumatic stress response. Most certainly humans weren't designed to endure high-speed collisions. Car bumpers are shock absorbers designed to withstand only minor impacts of five to ten miles per hour. In my own accident, the cumulative force was 110 miles per hour. Imagine the shock such an impact causes to your body.

Today we know a great deal more about treating the various levels of Post Traumatic Stress Response that occur as the result of accidents. We understand from our experience with war veterans, hostages, childhood abuse, earthquake victims, and other traumatic events that PTSD or PTSR is more than an emotional disturbance. It has a physical basis. Untreated, it can have lasting physical, emotional, and cognitive repercussions. Our goal is to help you put your life back together so that you aren't living your entire life with disabling symptoms.

Be assured that with this book, you can anticipate not only a lessening of symptoms, but also a new approach to both your accident and other life stresses. This will give you the power to cope and live a more fulfilling life by accessing resources your body already possesses.

Key Points

- Auto accidents affect more than 10 million people worldwide each year

- Auto accidents cause people to stay stuck in survival mode due to nervous system destabilization

- Survival mode causes physical and emotional symptoms, which may seem unrelated to the accident. These symptoms are not "in your head"

- Somatic Experiencing therapy and the Heller Resiliency Model offer relief for most symptoms

2

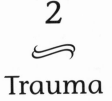

Trauma

What Is Trauma?

Trauma is perhaps the most avoided, ignored, belittled, denied, misunderstood, and untreated cause of human suffering. Although it is the source of tremendous distress and dysfunction, it is not an ailment or a disease, but the by-product of an instinctively instigated, altered state of consciousness. We enter this altered state—let us call it survival mode—when we perceive that our lives are being threatened. If we are overwhelmed by the threat and are unable to successfully defend ourselves, we can become stuck in survival mode. This highly aroused state is designed solely to enable short-term defensive actions; but left untreated over time, it begins to form the symptoms of trauma.

—Peter A. Levine, Ph.D.

Raymond B. Flannery, Jr., Ph.D., sums up the experience of trauma in his book, *Post-Traumatic Stress Disorder:* "Psychological trauma is the state of severe fright that we experience when we are confronted

> Definition: Trauma is any event that breaks the body's stimulus barrier, leading to overwhelming feelings of helplessness.

with a sudden, unexpected, potentially life-threatening event over which we have no control, and to which we are unable to respond effectively no matter how hard we try."

During an auto accident, there is too much stimulus to deal with at once. Think of being in a room with a radio turned up too loud and being unable to turn it off or move away from it. Events that might be manageable one at a time become overwhelming or traumatic when too many of them crowd in on us at once.

> *An experience is traumatic if it is: 1) Sudden, unexpected, non-normative, 2) Exceeds the individual's perceived ability to meet its demands.*
> —Lisa McCann, Ph.D.,
> in *Psychological Trauma and the Adult Survivor.*

Judith Lewis Herman, M.D., author of *Trauma and Recovery,* says:

> *Traumatic events are extraordinary not because they occur rarely, but rather because they overwhelm the ordinary human adaptations to life . . . the common denominator of psychological trauma is a feeling of "intense fear, helplessness, loss of control, and threat of annihilation."*

In Somatic Experiencing jargon, we say trauma is experiencing too much, too fast, too soon.

What Causes Trauma?

Trauma results from any event that overwhelms a person's capacity to cope. In this state of "overwhelm," a person experiences a fundamental "shutting down" that results in a loss of connection to self and others. It doesn't matter if someone else would be traumatized in that situation or not. Many people have felt shame about their own reactions or mystified by a friend or loved one's reaction to what seems like a minor traffic accident. You will come to understand why even seemingly small events can sometimes trigger significant trauma symptoms.

One of the reasons auto accidents can be so devastating is that they usually catch us by surprise. One minute we're driving along feeling fine, maybe listening to our favorite CD or talking with a friend; the next minute we may find ourselves waking up with paramedics standing over us.

Put yourself in this scenario: You're driving down the highway. Everything is fine. Suddenly, with no warning of danger, you hit a patch of black ice. You tighten your grip on the wheel. The car starts spinning. Oncoming traffic is a blur as your car careens out of control. You feel frozen, terrified, unable to take any action, only able to hope that you come out of this alive. Depending on the outcome and the person who experiences it, this kind of situation can result in trauma response and trauma symptoms.

People react differently to potentially traumatic situations. In the above scenario, if the car spins out and ends up safely at the side of the road, we might see a range of reactions. Some people, as soon as they realize they successfully escaped injury, would feel exhilarated and excited. Others may feel so much fear from the realization of what could have happened that they feel confused and disoriented, even after they land safely on the side of the road. In the future they may feel apprehensive or even phobic about driving on ice.

In a more tragic scenario the experience may have resulted in waking up in an emergency room and finding out a passenger or someone in the other car was killed—causing traumatization.

We see that some events would traumatize some people and not others, whereas more severe events would traumatize anyone. A person's reaction or capacity to cope in any specific event is influenced by what we call their Range of Resiliency as well as by the specifics of the event.

An individual's Range of Resiliency is in turn influenced by factors such as genetic background, personal history and current support system, and whether or not they have experienced other traumas in their life.

You can well imagine, for example, that if a person who just experienced a fender-bender had been in an accident five years prior where her passenger died, her reaction would likely be very different than that of someone who had never been in a previous accident.

Similarly, if a person's brother had been seriously injured in an accident three months prior, we might expect them to have more of a reaction than someone who doesn't have that experience. As we help you access and work through your own accident, it is important to take into consideration all the factors that affect your reaction to your accident.

In Chapter 3, we are going to give you a short course on how the body deals with danger. This is important for you to understand as you work on resolving your own auto accident trauma.

We're going to take you through the step by step process of how the body mobilizes to meet danger. Because of the suddenness and the sometimes high velocity involved, we often find ourselves out of control with no time to prepare or respond, no time for the usual fight-or-flight mechanisms to complete. You are strapped into a moving tin can. Your body mobilizes to meet threat, only to face total helplessness. Your brain, endocrine system, and nervous system are completely mobilized, but with you have no possibility to effectively respond. Having these powerful fight-or-flight energies activated in your body without the possibility of completing these reactions has long-term implications for both your mental and physical well-being—a phenomenon which until recently was little understood.

The following chapters are designed to first help you identify the various steps your body/mind goes through as it mobilizes to meet danger. Then we will clarify how the body may get stuck in survival mode in auto accidents. Finally, we will provide a step-by-step process to help you discharge the arousal that remains in your body when you get stuck in survival mode.

Key Points

- Trauma is anything that overwhelms a person's capacity to cope

- Many factors influence whether and how traumatic an event is for any given individual

- Traumatic events become a problem when we stay stuck in survival mode

- To heal trauma we have to learn how to discharge and complete the physical fight-or-flight energies that were mobilized to meet danger in order move out of survival mode

3

⤳

Trauma In Your Body

Threat Response

To help you understand what happens in your body when you face danger, envision the following scenario. As you do this, notice what happens in your body.

You're home alone at night in bed reading quietly. You hear a strange sound. You're startled. Examine what just happened in your body. Do you notice the feeling of muscles tightening? You hold your breath. You stop whatever you are doing. You are on total alert. You try to locate the danger, to identify the sound. You listen carefully. Where is it coming from? Your eyes fix on one spot as you listen, then they scan for danger. Notice what you experience in your body now.

You go to the window. Ah! It's just a tree branch scraping against the house. You sigh. Your muscles relax. You calmly get back in bed. Your eyes return to the book. But wait! There it is again—and it's not the tree branch. Your heart starts to race. You get goose bumps. Your breathing quickens. Muscles tense. All your senses are heightened. Your reptilian brain signals your body to mobilize its defenses. This is not something you do consciously. It's a biological response. Your fight-or-flight response has kicked in as the survival part of your brain prepares you to fight danger or run.

Suddenly a strange man hurtles into your bedroom. What do you do? So quickly that you are not aware of it, your survival brain assesses your three choices. If you are cornered, fighting the stranger may be your best option. If you are close to another door out of the room, flight may be your reflexive choice. If your brain's rapid assessment determines that you cannot successfully fight the intruder and you have no escape route, it may cause your body to freeze. You become immobile, unable to react.

Freeze is an ancient response of prey animals, a way to hide from the attacker. In the human hunter/hunted situation, freezing may reduce or de-escalate the attacker's level of violence. Many of us freeze during trauma because biologically it is one of our life-saving options.

When a body mobilizes its defenses in response to threat by either fighting, fleeing, or freezing, and then is unable to complete the response or to discharge those defensive energies, it is left in a state of overarousal and disequilibrium. If not resolved, there are far-reaching implications for our health and well-being.

> NOTE: Unfortunately many trauma survivors live with tremendous shame for having frozen in the face of danger when in actuality your body responded in the only way it knew how. When the *freeze* response occurs, it is a decision made by the reptilian brain as your best chance for survival in that situation. The fact that you are reading this is proof that it worked.

Why Understand the Threat Response?

The threat response is a predictable series of reactions governing how we respond physiologically to danger. Trauma, by definition, involves a sense of danger. You need to understand the sequence of the threat response in order to understand your natural reactions and where your body might get stuck or feel incomplete. After describing to you in detail how the body responds to threat we will show you how to move through the sequence successfully, which helps discharge the overarousal and return your nervous system to equilibrium.

Now let's look at what just happened to you in the above "home alone" scenario in terms of the threat response. Hearing the noise triggered a *startle response.* Your body starts undergoing profound physiological changes. You brace, your muscles contract. Breathing halts briefly or slows. Your nervous system becomes highly aroused. Your endocrine system is secreting powerful chemicals. This is all as nature designed it to be. Our body is preparing to meet the threat. We are preparing to fight or run.

You stopped what you were doing, an *arrest response,* and became very alert. Your field of vision narrowed. Your hearing became selective. Then you *scanned to locate the threat.* Your full attention was focused on evaluating the possible danger. Believing the noise was a tree branch, you *evaluated the source as non-threatening.* You slowly relaxed and returned to normal functioning. Feeling curious, you used your *exploratory orienting response* when your field of vision widened and you looked around. Returning to bed, you experienced a *relaxation response.* When the noise was repeated, you went through startle and arrest again, then experienced a *defensive orienting response.* As the stranger entered your room, your body chose a *fight, flight, or freeze response,* which are different categories of what we call a *defensive orienting response.* Your survival brain, in its best attempt to defend you, determined whether it was best to fight the threat or to avoid it by running away. If neither of these responses are possible because you are trapped or immobilized, you may experience a *freeze response,* in which people often report feeling cold, paralyzed, or unable to move. Often they feel disconnected or dissociated as well.

Symptoms When the Threat Response Sequence Has Not Been Completed

When our capacity to defend ourselves by running, fighting, or freezing is not successful, the unreleased survival energies stay stuck in our bodies. We stay in survival mode, where if a person stays for any extended period of time, they become symptomatic. These symptoms might include:

- Anxiety—Excessive Energy or Restlessness

- Feeling Disconnected

- Disorientation
- Fear or Helplessness
- Hypervigilance
- Sexual Apathy
- Constant Exhaustion
- Physical Pain
- Easily Startled
- Triggered by Similar Events
- Weight Gain

You may feel a loss of self, a sense of being dissociated, or in extreme cases a feeling of watching yourself from a distance. You lose your sense of safety and your trust in others. Feeling disoriented in time and space is common. People who are traumatized lose not only their connection to themselves, but to others. Because you find it hard to trust, you may push away those closest to you and become isolated.

Narrowed Choices

When the body tries something that doesn't work, the brain puts it in the "reject file." Your choices become so narrowed that you are at risk. As a result of early life traumas, you can get stuck in one survival strategy, usually fight, flight, or freeze. These choices are not made on a conscious level, but are the self-preservation part of the brain in action. Some adults may have learned early on that fighting was the only way to overcome neighborhood bullies, and may still confront unexpected situations with physical violence. Others may have learned that avoiding danger worked, and thus use flight as adults. Abused children who found there was no escape from their situations often live their lives in a freeze response. They become resigned and may collapse immediately when challenged.

Once choices are reinstated, the body will choose fight, flight, or freeze depending on current circumstances, instead of past conditioning. We are much safer with a full menu of options when faced with potential threat.

Our goal is to help you resolve your reaction to trauma so that you will have a full range of survival choices at your discretion. You can choose to use fight, flight, or freeze when you are threatened. And even more importantly, because you will no longer be in survival mode, you will not be hyperaroused, always expecting danger or something bad to happen.

How Nature Copes

It appears that animals in the wild, particularly prey animals such as rabbits and deer, despite facing continual threat, do not suffer from the after-effects of trauma. Why is this so, and what are the implications for humans?

When it comes to dealing with trauma, one advantage animals seem to have over humans is the lack of a highly developed neocortex, the higher reasoning aspect of the brain. Being less rational and more instinctive, they allow themselves to complete the normal sequence dictated by their nervous system to discharge arousal and return to equilibrium.

The following examples were developed by Dr. Peter Levine and have been explained in detail in his book on trauma, *Waking the Tiger: Healing Trauma*.

You may have seen a dog trying to cross a busy highway. As he crosses, he barely misses being hit by a car. He darts across the final lanes and collapses under a bush. To an observer, it looks as if he's been injured as he lies there, motionless. He has collapsed into a natural immobility response after a potentially near-death situation.

Gradually, movement begins to return, which is also a natural biological process. First, an eyelid flickers. His eyes open, and he looks around, moving only his eyes to orient himself to his surroundings. Meanwhile, his ears twitch, listening for danger. Next, his head slowly turns in an involuntary motion "as if his head is moving him versus him moving his head." Sensing no danger, he slowly stretches each limb as if testing them, perhaps scanning his body for injury.

He staggers to his feet. He begins to tremble, with the movement traveling from his head through his shoulders and haunches to the tip of his tail. As the shaking stops, he relaxes completely and trots jauntily off as if nothing has happened. His nervous system has taken the time it needed to re-establish equilibrium and release the excess energy. He knew instinctively to stop and wait for his nervous system to reorganize before exposing himself to further stimulation.

Another example Levine uses is that of a bird striking a window-pane because it doesn't recognize glass as a barrier. After impact the bird falls to the ground motionless, appearing dead. Then as you watch, small movement begins. First there are tiny eye movements, then orienting movements with the neck to "locate itself." It begins to shake and flutter its wings erratically. If uninjured, the wings coordinate and eventually the bird recovers and flies away.

What happens if you pick the bird up before it can fly? You may be trying to help but unfortunately you are interrupting an important physiological process. Often the bird goes back into the motionless state, going even deeper into shock. It can actually die from terror. Interrupting the cycle is dangerous and harmful. In accidents, humans are almost always interrupted after shocks—dealing with the other driver, police reports, and getting back to work as soon as possible.

As Levine says, "Unfortunately, humans have a much harder time completing this process. There are two main reasons for this difficulty. One, the survival energy is so intense that it frightens us; and two, we are uncomfortable with surrendering our conscious control to involuntary (unconscious) sensations. Because of these fears, our rational brains often try to override the completion process. When this happens, the nervous system remains in a state of arousal. Even if the threat is gone, brain and body respond as if it still exists and continue to spew out the fight-or-flight chemicals."

An accident or trauma creates a tremendous energy response in the body. The natural or instinctual urge is to aggressively confront the threat or run from it—the fight-or-flight response. There's a burst of adrenaline and other biochemical reactions and the body is ready for action. When it's totally overwhelmed or blocked the body freezes, trapping all that mobilized survival energy.

That undischarged survival energy in the nervous system, we believe, is the source of most of the symptoms commonly recognized as PTSD. Helping you learn how to recognize and discharge this survival energy will be the focus of Chapter 5.

First we want to talk a little more about the brain. We mentioned previously how the lack of a highly developed neo-cortex helps animals avoid the long-term effects of trauma. Next we are going to briefly explain the biology of the brain and how we can use this understanding of our brains to help ourselves heal from trauma.

Key Points

- The threat response has a predictable sequence

- Humans deal with threat in three ways—fight, flight, or freeze

- These defensive responses mobilize a great deal of energy

- Long-term trauma symptoms develop when these survival energies remain locked in our bodies and are not resolved or completed

4

∽

How Your Brain Works

Our brain has three levels that work together in an integrated way, though each level has a dominant function. This is often called the "triune brain." The level that makes us uniquely human is the neo-cortex, also known as the neo-mammalian or cognitive brain. It's the part that is thinking, creative, and makes us individuals. It is closely related to what we call the conscious mind.

A deeper level of our brain is the limbic or paleo-mammalian brain, responsible for emotions and feelings. An even deeper level is what's known as the reptilian or "primitive" brain that includes your brain stem. Evolutionarily speaking, it's the oldest part of the brain, an expert on survival. It's in charge of all the involuntary functions—sleeping, appetite, breathing, heart rate, perspiration, temperature regulation, and sexual function, as well as self-preservation and reproduction.

Because the reptilian brain is in charge of survival, it's the part that automatically takes over when you feel threatened. This part of the brain controls what we have called the defensive orienting response, the well known fight-or-flight response, as well as the freeze response which we will explain in this chapter. In an auto accident the reptilian brain is in control—and that's exactly how it has evolved to function. In traumatic events when our fight-or-flight mechanism becomes highly mobilized, but ends up being overwhelmed and ineffective, it is this part of the brain and the evolutionary function controlled by it that are the most affected.

Think about your trauma symptoms and about the involuntary functions that we're discussing. Do you see a relationship here? Since your accident you may be having trouble sleeping or you may have lost interest in sex. Perhaps you've gained or lost weight. Some people find themselves hyperventilating or experiencing shallow breathing. Others experience digestive upsets. Your heart may sometimes race and you may have strange temperature shifts. All of these involuntary physiological functions are controlled by the reptilian brain.

Let's try and understand the fight-or-flight mechanism through the use of an analogy. The fight-or-flight mechanism is controlled in the sympathetic branch of the autonomic nervous system. Simply put, the sympathetic part of the nervous system has to do with charging the system, giving us energy. It's like the gas pedal of our nervous system. In normal life it is the energy from this branch of the nervous system that gears up to help us get our needs met, pursue our dreams, and accomplish our goals.

The parasympathetic branch, on the other hand, is more like the brake pedal of our nervous system. It helps to discharge the arousal generated by the sympathetic branch and move us back into relaxation. This branch fuels the sense of relaxation we feel after a good day's work, or after a goal has been met.

Under normal conditions there is a gentle rhythm between the two consisting of charge and discharge. When that rhythm is in place, we experience a sense of well-being and life feels manageable.

Resilient Nervous System

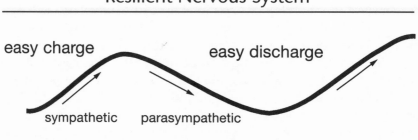

easy charge   easy discharge

sympathetic   parasympathetic

Two Types of Trauma Reaction

A person experiencing the freeze response on the surface may look normal and calm. Let's go back to the comparison of the sympathetic nervous system as your car's gas pedal, and the parasympathetic as the brakes: you realize that a person in freeze response has pressed the accelerator to the floor while simultaneously jamming on the brakes, so that the engine is fully engaged but the car can't budge. Of course, you wouldn't ever want to treat your car this way.

This dramatic example of how NOT to drive a car accurately reflects the situation inside your body when the autonomic nervous system is deregulated. The sympathetic branch is fully engaged to mobilize massive amounts of survival energy to help you defend yourself in the face of danger or threat. The parasympathetic branch has the brakes on attempting to control the mobilization. You may feel alternating flooding of excess energy in the form of a racing heart, excessive sweating, angry outbursts or panic attacks, and symptoms of shutting down, such as fatigue, disconnection, or depression. Inside, just like the mistreated automobile, your system is reacting as if you were pressing down hard on both the accelerator and the brakes of your car simultaneously. If others could see inside you, they would see that your engine is racing, while the brakes are holding you back. It consumes a tremendous amount of energy. When the nervous system is deregulated you cannot avoid feeling exhausted!

Exercise: You Can't NOT Be Tired!

This exercise will show you how exhausting these two opposing forces can be.

Push your hands against one another as hard as you can. Keep pushing. From a distance, an observer might see you with your hands together and believe you are relaxed in prayer. But up close, it becomes evident how much energy you are exerting in this "deadlocked" position.

If you push hard enough, your hands and arms may begin to tremble. Feel how much energy you are using! You can't release just one hand. Both have to give gently.

Feel how tired you are when you release the pressure? Fatigue goes along with the energy exerted to maintain these opposing forces.

Let's use a different analogy to describe what happens to our nervous system when facing a traumatic life experience that is overwhelming, like many automobile accidents. Compare your nervous system to your house's electrical system: What happens if you run 220 volts through a 110-volt system? In modern houses the breakers switch off to protect the system. This is analogous to the dissociation or disconnection from self that happens when a human being is overloaded in a traumatic event. Many trauma victims describe themselves as having had their circuits blown. Others feel like their nerve endings have been "fried." Obviously the breakers switch off to protect the wiring of the home from burning up. In the same way, people dissociate or disconnect to protect themselves from the devastation of trauma.

Many therapists, when seeing that a person is disconnected or out of touch with her body and not feeling, try to get the patient to "reconnect" and start feeling again. If this is not done slowly, as we are proposing, often what happens is similar to switching the electrical breakers back on without doing something about the overload that caused the breaker to go off in the first place. When therapists get a client to connect too quickly, they can often retraumatize them. Our approach employs techniques to drain the overload out of a person's system so that they can reconnect gradually and relatively painlessly.

What happens in the body and the nervous system as a result of trauma is so important for you to comprehend that we want to offer another analogy. Let's describe what happens in trauma using the flooding/freezing/flooding analogy.

In traumatic events it is as if a person is being flooded by stimuli. As one of our clients, a former surfer, described his accident: "It happened so fast I felt like I was riding the biggest out-of-control wave of my life and it was throwing me straight at the rocks with nothing I could do about it." Another client described her accident: "All of a sudden I felt like I was watching ten TV channels simultaneously and couldn't focus clearly on any one of them."

A person feels inundated with fear, helplessness, and other powerful emotions. She responds by freezing her body and her nervous system. Think about how we describe ourselves or others as "scared stiff" or "frozen with fear." This freezing is protective and actually part of a biological defense mechanism, like a deer in the headlights. Prey animals have used freezing for millennia to avoid predators.

When people get stuck in freeze response, however, they may experience disconnection, a feeling of deadness, meaninglessness, depression, and dissociation.

After trauma, people may go back and forth between flooding and freezing, a vicious and painful cycle. Triggers associated with the traumatic event can take a person from freezing to flooding. In the flooding state that comes after a traumatic event, a person may experience panic, rage, flashbacks, or other symptoms we have described. Therapies that move too quickly can also cause flooding. A person needs to move out of the frozen state back to aliveness. But this unfreezing needs to be done slowly, one step at a time, so

Overactivated Nervous System

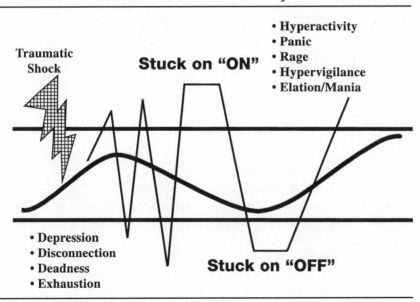

that a person can integrate the experience back into her life, moving from freezing back into the flow of life.

Fight, Flight, and Freeze

In auto accidents, you may attempt flight by trying to get out of the way if you have enough warning. However, when you are confined in a car, fight-or-flight is usually impossible, so freeze may be the natural response to an accident. Many times, accident or trauma victims blame themselves afterwards for taking no action. It's important that you understand this was an unconscious decision made for you by your reptilian brain that perceived freezing as your best bet for survival.

When terror or anxiety continue to persist as symptoms afterward, this usually indicates the presence of an incomplete flight response. When rage and anger persist as symptoms, it often signals an incomplete fight response. Both fight and flight responses need to be completed on a physiological level for the stored hyperarousal to be effectively discharged, allowing the body to truly relax. The freeze response may overlay symptoms from thwarted fight-or-flight reactions that emerge in the aftermath of an accident. An unresolved freeze response can inhibit the possibility for a person to take action to protect themselves in future dangerous situations.

Amy

The following story illustrates the importance of relaxing the freeze response in order not to be more vulnerable to future accidents.

When Amy had her first rear-end accident, she was crowded in by other cars. The truck approached so rapidly that there was no way for her to avoid the collision. At the time of her second accident, she saw the vehicle approaching her from behind well in advance. She realized it couldn't stop. Though the intersection ahead of her was clear, and she might have avoided the accident by moving her car, she immediately froze.

During the first accident, Amy had no choice in how to react. There wasn't time or space. Because she was not yet recovered at the time of the second accident, she was unable to make any choice but to freeze even when she could have protected herself. Her nervous system was so overwhelmed that her brain's response was immobility. Her original response of uncontrollable freezing was re-evoked even though she had a choice to avoid collision.

In treatment, Amy learned how to complete the freeze response and to reinstate fight and flight possibilities by rehearsing them and feeling them in her body. She gained a much broader range of responses and is now much safer when she drives.

The techniques in this book will help you release your frozen energy gradually, bit by bit, until you can tolerate more energy. The techniques of looping between resources and the events of your accident we describe in Chapters 6 and 7 will help you tremendously as you work to gradually release the tension. Remember, our mottoes are "slower is faster" and "less is more."

Getting the Shakes Is a Good Sign

When the event is over, you may find you are trembling uncontrollably, as did the dog or bird following stress. The shaking or trembling is the body's way of releasing the trapped excess energy. Once the body has rested, then released its energy, it returns to a normal energy baseline. The autonomic nervous system can then re-regulate and involuntary functioning can normalize. Normal sleep patterns replace chronic sleep disturbance or avoidance of feelings manifested by oversleeping. Appetite becomes regular and over- or under-eating is no longer a problem. Emotions even out and are realistically responsive to current circumstances. Fear and anger subside and are no longer constant companions. You feel like it is safe to live in your body again and feel reconnected to your body, your sense of self, and your significant others. You no longer feel shame or the need to isolate and can begin to accept support. As Levine points out, *"When animals determine that they are not in danger, they often begin to vibrate, twitch, and lightly tremble.... These little tremblings of muscular tissue are the organism's way of regulating extremely different stages of nervous system activation."*

35

NOTE: Trembling is a good sign. It signals that your excess energy is being released. It is an involuntary response you cannot control. We recommend you allow it to continue.

If you begin trembling at any stage during this work, it is a very good sign, though it may feel strange and uncomfortable. The shaking and trembling moves you from fixity, the frozen state, back into flow, the natural state of a regulated nervous system. Think of a block of ice gradually thawing into a flowing stream. We want to bring your system out of freeze response gradually.

Trembling is a sign that your nervous system is unwinding. It's the state we are hoping to evoke. Let it continue as long as you are able, taking a break if necessary. Afterward, you may feel tired because the energy released is intense, but you should experience a strong sense of well-being, as well as the capacity to relax more deeply.

How the Impact May Thwart Natural Discharge

Reading this material requires concentration and we suggest you read it at home or in a comfortable place where there are no distractions. If you feel distracted, even by your own car accident memories while reviewing the material, take a break. We recommend you take a break after each exercise, as well as every 30 to 45 minutes of reading, or turn to the chapter on resources and do the first exercise.

During a car accident, we're trapped in the mobile equivalent of a tin can. We're usually strapped into a seatbelt. We can't fight. There's nowhere to run. Immediately after the accident, we have to cope with all sorts of outside stimuli and demands. There may be emergency personnel or police asking questions. There are accident reports and insurance forms to fill out. There's an immediate need to call our boss or our family—not to mention the worry about our wrecked car and how we're going to get it repaired.

All this extra stimulation comes on top of a life-threatening event, at the very time our body is demanding that we "crawl under a bush" and remain quiet and still until we're ready to dissipate the extra energy. Instead, we're like the bird picked up before it recovers. Our process is interrupted and the excess energy created at the time of the accident is literally trapped inside us. Our fight-or-flight response doesn't get completed and continues to cycle within us, building on itself. Our capacity to discharge is compromised or unavailable.

This trapped energy makes the reptilian brain think the threat is still present. It reacts as it is programmed to do, by shutting off as much outside stimulus as possible or by feeling uncontrollably flooded by stimulus. Trapped stimulus and incomplete natural physiological responses cause the symptoms of trauma you're experiencing. This is a point that cannot be stressed too strongly. In Somatic Experiencing we say, "trauma is in the body, not in the event." It means that although the original event was external to us, what causes trauma symptoms is the overload of energy experienced in the body. The mind experiences the overload as threatening, and without realizing it projects the danger outward as if the threat were external or yet to happen.

Understanding this principle helps a person who experienced trauma come to terms with the sense of dread, or "waiting for the other shoe to fall" that is often experienced after a person has been traumatized.

Getting in Touch with the Reptilian Brain

Healing trauma is accomplished by doing everything in reverse, but in a controlled way. You work back through the trauma piece by piece, but not in the same sequence as the original events. *Remember that it is very important that you work through the experience nonsequentially.* It is important to insert lots of extra time between segments to allow your body to develop the awareness of what it needs or would have done if there simply had been more time. In car accidents, even seconds make a huge difference.

The first step is learning how to get in touch with your reptilian brain. That's difficult for us, because ours is not a physically aware culture. We're proud of our cognitive abilities, our ability to convince ourselves intellectually that there's nothing wrong with us. But as you have noticed, the reptilian brain isn't convinced by these messages from the cognitive brain.

Our neocortex specializes in abstract thinking and our reptilian brain specializes in self-preservation. Our reptilian brain has centuries of experience behind it to draw upon, which is why it is the expert in survival strategies.

The reptilian brain is very basic and processes information slowly. It deals in sensation, imagery, and metaphors. It likes stories. Because the reptilian brain processes information much more slowly than the cognitive brain, we must speak to it slowly and simply. Don't try to impress the reptilian brain with your vocabulary! Keep the language simple.

Sensation language—touch, taste, sound, smell, and sight—appeals to the reptilian brain. This isn't what we're used to hearing from one another. It's not the way we interact. We have to learn to "speak sensation" to contact and stay connected with the reptilian brain. It is like learning a foreign language. At first, you have to convert from English to French or German consciously. Eventually you become more fluent and you think in German or French without having to translate. Be careful not to ask yourself questions such as "What do I think?" These questions access your neocortex rather than the reptilian brain, which deals predominantly with sensation.

We're going to take you through a dialogue Larry used when working with a client. It shows how we work with sensation in the body. Once you have read the chapter on resourcing refer back to this dialogue to help you understand how we use positive states in the body as resources.

Larry converses with Marta, who was experiencing chronic pain throughout her body after her traffic accident six months earlier:

L: *How are you feeling?*
M: *Terrible, as usual. Everything hurts.*
L: *I know it feels like everything hurts, but try an internal scan of your body and see if you can feel any place that doesn't hurt.*
M: *Well actually, I'm surprised to see that my hands don't hurt.*
L: *Great! Let's explore the feeling in your hands for a moment. You say they don't hurt. What do they feel like? Take your time to check it out.*
M: *They are warm and they feel kind of soft.*

L: They are warm and they feel soft.

M: Yeah.

L: See what happens if you give yourself time to experience the warmth and the softness in your hands.

M: Well, when I bring my attention there, my hands get even warmer and start to tingle a little.

L: And as you pay attention to the warmth, the softness and the tingling, what else do you notice?

M: Well, actually, the warmth starts to move up my arms.

L: Very good. And as you continue to pay attention to that warmth that is now moving up your arms, what happens next?

M: Well strangely, my arms are relaxing even more, all the way up to the kinks in my neck. This is so surprising!

L: With a little help, your body knows what to do. Describe the kinks in your neck to me.

M: They are like painful knots.

L: Is there a temperature to the knots?

M: Now that you ask, they feel kind of cold.

L: Bring your awareness back to your arms. What are you experiencing there right now?

M: They are still warm and relaxed. I'm sure they were hurting when I came in.

L: Your arms are still warm and relaxed. Now bring your awareness back to the kinks in your neck.

M: They feel a little different.

L: In what way?

M: It's hard to describe. Maybe not quite so tight.

L: Now go back to your arms. What's happening there?

M: They are still warm and tingly.

L: Anything else you notice?

M: Well, that tingly feeling is moving into my neck a little bit. It's what is softening the kinks.

L: I'm going to have you go back and forth between the warmth and tingling in your arms and the kinks in your neck. First focus for a moment on your arms and what you are feeling there. Now go for just a moment to the kinks in your neck. Now back to your arms.

(This looping back and forth is continued for several minutes.)

L: Now what are you aware of in your arms and neck?

M: The kinks aren't completely gone, but they are much less intense and warmer. Should I try and relax them some more?

L: Notice, in the exercise we were doing you weren't trying to relax anything. Trying to relax often makes things tighter.

M: What should I do then?

L: Just continue to pay attention to what's happening in your arms and neck.

Pain is often a magnet that keeps our awareness captive. Larry helped Marta find a positive pain-free resource in her body. Bringing her awareness to it, it began to expand by itself. The response expanded by itself until it bumped into the activation in Marta's neck. By looping back and forth between the resource (the warmth in her hands and then arms), the activation (constriction and knots in her neck), and focusing on sensation, the tension in her neck began to dissolve.

Exercise: Speaking Sensation Language

The goal of this exercise is to help you learn to "speak sensation."

You see a beautiful sunset. You say to yourself, "This is great." It's so beautiful, you take it a step further for three times the effect. Ask yourself "What do I feel in my body when I see those vivid colors, the mountains, the light breaking through the clouds?" You may feel warm and tingly, the beginning of pleasure—an expansion in your chest, an opening in your heart, and a sense of love for life. You have just begun to feel grounded in your body's sensations.

Sensation Language

Finding words to describe physical sensations can be difficult because we don't often describe our experience that way. When a friend asks us how we are, we may say "fine" but probably don't say, "Well, I feel expanded in my chest, a little tight in my neck and a bit cold in my lower legs." Here is a partial list of "sensation" terms:

Dense	Thick	Flowing
Breathless	Fluttery	Nervous
Queasy	Expanded	Floating
Heavy	Tingly	Electric
Fluid	Numb	Wooden
Dizzy	Full	Congested
Spacey	Trembly	Twitchy
Tight	Hot	Bubbly
Achy	Wobbly	Itchy
Frozen	Shaky	Calm
Suffocating	Buzzy	Energized
Contracted	Expansive	Smooth
Tremulous	Constricted	Warm
Knotted	Icy	Light
Blocked	Hollow	Cold
Disconnected	Sweaty	Streaming

This sensation language is so foreign to the way we usually think or speak that you may find it hard to accept until you have tried some of the exercises I suggest. Give your reptilian brain a chance to show you the power of your body's natural ability to heal!

Exercise: Contacting Your Reptilian Brain

The goal of this exercise is to practice getting in touch with your reptilian brain.

Sit in a comfortable chair. As you start to read this, take a moment to scan your body. You may want to close your eyes for a few minutes to focus inward and bring awareness into your body. Where do you feel the most support physically? Feel your backside on the seat of the chair. Feel your arms on the arms of the chair. Sense the weight of your feet on the floor. Notice how your clothing feels against your skin.

Just take a few moments to sense how and where your body feels supported. Let yourself relax into being supported there if possible. Is it comfortable? Pleasant? How does it feel to have your feet on the floor? If you are having trouble feeling your feet, press them gently against the floor.

Gradually increase the pressure. This helps bring back feeling. Just let yourself sit and feel for a few minutes. Bring your awareness to your physical sensations. Do an internal scan of the physical sensations in your body at this moment. Go slowly. Don't judge, analyze, or try to change anything. Just take a physical inventory.

You might notice areas of tension or constriction you are feeling in your body. Does the tension have a size or shape? Do you sense that it has a color or a density? Don't do anything about the tension now. Just notice and be aware. Notice where your body feels most comfortable. Notice where it feels warm or cool. Do you notice a tingling sensation anywhere?

This exercise is usually very relaxing and reassuring. The very act of paying attention to your body changes your experience. It helps you feel connected. It's a good starting point for the next steps in our work. If your awareness seems less embodied, in other words, you feel disconnected from your body, just notice what you are experiencing from your current perspective. For instance, if you feel you are observing events from above your body instead of from inside it, then track your experience from wherever that place is. As you work, your awareness and sense of connectedness will increase.

Exercise 1: Regaining Sensation

Here is another exercise, suggested by Peter Levine for regaining sensation:

Get a pulsating showerhead for your shower. As you are showering, notice how the water feels on your body. Change the settings, and notice the difference. You also can sit in a hot tub and vary the pressure from the jets for a similar effect. Just a slight change in temperature or water pressure can be more or less pleasurable. How does it feel? Is it pleasant, or unpleasant? Does your body like the feeling? What temperature is the most pleasing to you?

Levine also suggests going to a gym and using the exercise equipment to be more fully aware of your muscles and how they feel while working and then relaxing.

Many more techniques to focus on sensation are described in

Eugene Gendlin's book, *Focusing.* You will find an entire series of exercises to help you focus physically and listen to your body.

Exercise 2: Regaining Sensation and a Sense of Safety

This exercise helps you feel sensation in your body.

Think of a favorite place or time when you felt very safe, secure, and happy. What happens in your body when you imagine going there? Now, in your mind's eye, look around your favorite place. What do you see? Are there other people or are you alone? Are there sounds, colors, or temperatures associated with this time and place? What do you like about it there? What do you notice in your body as you remember this time and place where you felt safe, secure, and happy? How do you notice the feeling of safety in your body? Where in your body does this sense of safety register?

Feeling Sensation in Your Body

It's not enough just to think about your senses. The benefit comes when you actually feel the sensation in your body, noticing it as a physical experience.

You're exploring a whole new range of language here. What goes into the actual experience of "feeling good" is a range of overt and subtle sensations that, when interpreted by the brain, come together to indicate the whole impression of a good feeling. Accessing the reptilian brain involves distinguishing these discrete sensations, focusing on them, and allowing ourselves to feel them in a more conscious way. We might notice that we're feeling a pleasant tingling in our left arm and torso, that there's a good feeling of warmth and expansion in our chest, and that our neck feels relaxed. All these experiences together tell us we're feeling good.

In the same way, "feeling bad" encompasses a range of sensations. For instance, a stomach ache may involve feelings of compression, "butterflies," pressure, nausea, or feel like rocks or knots. Sometimes just identifying the specific feeling helps alleviate it because you are increasing your awareness there.

Normally, sensations are constantly changing and flowing. When a sensation is constant or fixed, like chronic pain or recurring anxiety, it's often a symptom of trauma and indicates trapped or bound activation that needs to be resolved.

In the chapter on Resourcing, you'll find more exercises to help you contact your reptilian brain and let your body release its trapped energy.

Exercise: Converting Thoughts, Images, Behaviors, and Feelings into Sensation

This exercise helps you convert thought and emotion into sensation. Think of it as "tunneling" back through the levels of your brain into the constant river of sensation in your body. To resolve trauma, you need a way to tap into your sensation and reach the reptilian brain.

Thoughts: *What happens when you have one of those self-critical thoughts, like "It was my fault because I'm stupid"? What happens in your body? You may feel weak, collapsed, constricted, or small like a child.*

Remember a time when you felt competent and confident, even powerful. What do you feel? Now take it one level further into sensation. You may feel strength in your body, well-grounded in your feet, an expansion in your chest, or a physical readiness to take on a challenge.

Emotion: *Remember a feeling of fear. How does your body show you that it's feeling fear physically? Some people say that they feel cold, their breathing becomes shallow or they feel breathless, their heart rate increases, or they feel constricted, paralyzed, or unable to think in an organized way.*

Images: *Do you notice a certain recurring image associated with the accident? What do you feel in your body when you see that image? Imagine an opposite image? What do you feel in your body when you see the opposite?*

Behaviors: *In a session I might say to you, "I keep seeing you swinging your leg or tapping your foot when we talk about the accident. What do you notice when you become aware of your foot moving? Do you get a sense of what it may be preparing to do?" One client, noticing this movement, realized she wanted to jam on the brake, to stop her car and avoid the crash. Notice if you have any restless movements that occur when talking about your accident.*

Feelings: *Identify another feeling state. For example, notice what happens when you feel loved, protected, and safe. What does that feel like in your body? You may feel relaxed, warm, cozy, a feeling of being held, supported, or comforted. Take your time with this. Both positive and negative states engaging thoughts, emotions, and images need to be experienced as physical sensations to release the trapped energy.*

Don't worry if you're having trouble with these exercises. It's important to be easy on yourself as you go back to sensation language. It's not something you've been trained to do, but you can learn awareness of sensation. Your trauma can make you feel so disconnected from your body that it may take some time to get back into yourself. Don't push yourself. If you're out of touch with your body, there's usually a reason. It's simply a sign of high activation, a natural result of overwhelming or traumatic events.

Key Points

- Survival and the fight-or-flight mechanism are regulated by the instinctive part of our brain, the so-called "reptilian brain"

- Trauma interrupts the normal easy flow of charge and discharge in the autonomic nervous system

- Trauma is like running 220 volts through a 110 volt system

- Common reactions after trauma include flooding and freezing

- Flooding symptoms include anxiety attacks, anger outbursts, and flashbacks

- Freezing symptoms include constriction, numbness, disconnection, dissociation, and immobility

5

Symptoms of Trauma

Assess the severity of your symptoms since the traumatic event with this chart. "0" means no difficulty or no negative impact on you, while "5" is extreme difficulty, a high level of interference in your life.

Trauma Symptom Survey

1.	Feelings of helplessness and/or powerlessness	0	1	2	3	4	5
2.	Lack of focus or concentration	0	1	2	3	4	5
3.	Gaps in memory—especially related to traumatic events	0	1	2	3	4	5
4.	Disorientation—confused about time, space, direction	0	1	2	3	4	5
5.	Prone to accident	0	1	2	3	4	5
6.	Feeling out of control	0	1	2	3	4	5
7.	Feeling frozen, paralyzed, immobile	0	1	2	3	4	5

8. Recurring dreams related
   to traumatic event   0   1   2   3   4   5

9. Intrusive imagery related
   to traumatic event, i.e. you
   can't stop seeing the accident   0   1   2   3   4   5

10. Flashbacks that make you feel
    you are reliving the accident   0   1   2   3   4   5

11. Disrupted sleeping patterns
    (circle one)
    insomnia oversleeping both   0   1   2   3   4   5

12. Lethargy, exhaustion,
    chronic fatigue   0   1   2   3   4   5

13. Night terrors or abrupt
    awakening with intense fear   0   1   2   3   4   5

14. Extreme emotional shifts   0   1   2   3   4   5

15. Rage or anger outbursts   0   1   2   3   4   5

16. overcautiousness   0   1   2   3   4   5

17. Fear of being watched
    or followed   0   1   2   3   4   5

18. Startle easily or "jumpy"   0   1   2   3   4   5

19. Feeling overwhelmed   0   1   2   3   4   5

20. Feeling defeated, inadequate,
    can't do anything   0   1   2   3   4   5

21. Feeling confused or fragmented   0   1   2   3   4   5

22. Too much energy (hyperactivity) 0   1   2   3   4   5

23. Impulses to run away
    or escape fantasies   0   1   2   3   4   5

24. Unable to feel weight of body,
    feeling outside of yourself   0   1   2   3   4   5

25. Feeling physically heavy, like
    dead weight   0   1   2   3   4   5

26. Losing personal items, such as
    keys, glasses, etc.   0   1   2   3   4   5

27. Feeling disconnected, lost,
    "not here"   0   1   2   3   4   5

28. Trouble keeping track of time,
    late for appointments   0   1   2   3   4   5

29. Trouble orienting in space, i.e.
    bumping into things   0   1   2   3   4   5

30. Avoidance of triggers
    or associations with event,
    i.e. fear of driving
    on the highway   0   1   2   3   4   5

31. Panic attacks   0   1   2   3   4   5

32. Feeling anxious   0   1   2   3   4   5

33. Nausea or vomiting   0   1   2   3   4   5

34. Shame   0   1   2   3   4   5

35. Self-judgment or self-blaming   0   1   2   3   4   5

36. Electric or overcharged
feeling in body   0 1 2 3 4 5

37. Obsessive review of incident,
constantly retelling the story. 0 1 2 3 4 5

38. Disrupted eating patterns
(Circle one)
over-eating under-eating both 0 1 2 3 4 5

39. Easily distracted 0 1 2 3 4 5

40. Chronic pain 0 1 2 3 4 5

41. Hypervigilance or
feeling "on guard" 0 1 2 3 4 5

42. Inability to cope
with normal stresses 0 1 2 3 4 5

43. Isolation from people 0 1 2 3 4 5

44. Constriction, suppression,
feeling shut down 0 1 2 3 4 5

45. Distrust 0 1 2 3 4 5

46. Little or no awareness
of choices 0 1 2 3 4 5

47. Disinterest in life 0 1 2 3 4 5

48. Generalized fear or anger, i.e.
believing all drivers are unsafe 0 1 2 3 4 5

49. Excessive worrying 0 1 2 3 4 5

50. Disrupted relationships	0	1	2	3	4	5
51. Alienation, believing no one can understand	0	1	2	3	4	5
52. Bonding with others through trauma	0	1	2	3	4	5
53. Sudden fearfulness for no apparent reason	0	1	2	3	4	5
54. Fearlessness of dangerous situations	0	1	2	3	4	5
55. Uncontrolled temper	0	1	2	3	4	5
56. Desire to hurt self or others	0	1	2	3	4	5
57. Loss of sexual interest	0	1	2	3	4	5
58. Dizziness	0	1	2	3	4	5
59. Idea that someone can control your thoughts	0	1	2	3	4	5
60. Fear of being alone	0	1	2	3	4	5
61. Fear of being with others	0	1	2	3	4	5
62. Crying easily	0	1	2	3	4	5
63. Inability to cry	0	1	2	3	4	5
64. Fear of leaving home or familiar surroundings	0	1	2	3	4	5

65.	"Everything's fine" stance	0	1	2	3	4	5
66.	No sense of future	0	1	2	3	4	5
67.	Loss of creativity	0	1	2	3	4	5
68.	Depression	0	1	2	3	4	5
69.	Shakiness	0	1	2	3	4	5
70.	Apathy, no energy for life	0	1	2	3	4	5
71.	Feeling dead or in "no man's land"	0	1	2	3	4	5
72.	Difficulty with starting projects	0	1	2	3	4	5
73.	Starting many projects and not completing them	0	1	2	3	4	5
74.	Hypersensitivity to sound or light	0	1	2	3	4	5
75.	Get feelings hurt easily	0	1	2	3	4	5
76.	Irritability, overreacting to things	0	1	2	3	4	5
77.	Compulsively rechecking everything you do	0	1	2	3	4	5
78.	Acting out (circle those that apply) throwing objects, screaming hitting or kicking, shouting	0	1	2	3	4	5
79.	Everything seems burdensome or daunting	0	1	2	3	4	5

80. Feeling weak in body, collapsed in joints	0	1	2	3	4	5
81. Feeling doomed, as if something bad is going to happen	0	1	2	3	4	5
82. Restlessness, can't settle	0	1	2	3	4	5
83. Heart pounding, racing, or irregular	0	1	2	3	4	5
84. Not remembering aspects of traumatic event	0	1	2	3	4	5
85. Difficulty connecting or feeling close to others	0	1	2	3	4	5
86. Difficulty making decisions	0	1	2	3	4	5
87. Guilt, regret, shame	0	1	2	3	4	5
88. Numbing, deadening of feeling or sensation	0	1	2	3	4	5
89. Stomach problems, nausea, upset, knots	0	1	2	3	4	5
90. Feelings of worthlessness, inadequacy	0	1	2	3	4	5
91. Feeling your life is still threatened	0	1	2	3	4	5
92. Increased urinary frequency	0	1	2	3	4	5
93. Temperature shifts— chills or hot flashes	0	1	2	3	4	5

94. Futurized memory or the dread trauma will occur	0	1	2	3	4	5
95. Feeling violated or unsafe	0	1	2	3	4	5
96. Emotional flooding (unable to control emotions)	0	1	2	3	4	5
97. Feeling heightened sense of urgency	0	1	2	3	4	5
98. Obsessive thinking about the accident	0	1	2	3	4	5
99. Sense of horror as witness to traumatic events	0	1	2	3	4	5
100. Feeling your life is in danger since the traumatic event(s)	0	1	2	3	4	5

Highlight the symptoms you marked 3, 4, or 5. These scores indicate moderate to severe difficulties that require more immediate attention. When you have several high scores, you may want to seek additional professional help. It is useful to take this symptom survey again periodically to evaluate your progress.

Sam

Though it isn't an automobile accident case, this case illustrates how trauma affects the reptilian brain, which in turn affects so much of our physiology, and shows how symptoms relate to trauma.

Sam, a psychotherapist, had been in a serious earthquake at 4:30 a.m. One minute he and his wife were sleeping peacefully. The next instant he was thrown from his bed and found himself on the floor in his bedroom with plaster and furniture raining down around him. It was pitch dark. He didn't know exactly where he was or even where his wife or children were. Fortunately, they all miraculously escaped uninjured, though the house was in shambles.

In a class I was teaching on trauma, Sam began telling about his experience. He insisted he had no after-effects from the earthquake. Further questioning revealed, however, that he had suffered an unusual number of respiratory infections in the year since the earthquake and had a nagging digestive problem that wasn't responding to medical treatment.

I suggested we do a bit of work to see if there was any remaining trauma and if these seemingly unrelated symptoms might be related to the earthquake. As he went back through the unsettling experience, he began to gasp for breath and feel constriction and burning in his lungs. He was so afraid when we revisited aspects of his earthquake experience that he experienced difficulty breathing, which is a common trauma symptom. Although breathing was not a problem in his everyday life, the respiratory ailment was a clue that there was unresolved activation. I helped him become calmer by going more slowly through his traumatic event.

I spent a lot of time helping his body slowly feel the shift from sleeping in a prone position to being harshly awakened and thrown upright and then down to the floor. I reminded him that he had survived the chaos and that his wife and children were safe. I had him visualize his wife and children and see how they are now, healthy and safe, until his body registered that fact and relaxed. Now he was freer to focus on himself and his own physiological reactions.

We spent time on how he had escaped and the relief he felt when the earthquake ceased. Gradually he was able to feel more grounded—especially important in reference to an earthquake experience where the ground itself feels lost or threatening. His breathing became fuller and easier.

We worked together to help his system discharge the excess energy and relax. I helped him locate and complete unfinished survival responses that he had not had the time to complete in the original circumstances. As we worked, he felt increasing relief and began to breathe much more easily. He began to see quite clearly that there was a direct connection between the earthquake and his respiratory ailments.

As we continued working, he was stricken with severe stomach pains. I worked with him by having him remember the deeper arousal that was the source of his stomach pain. I provided him with resources and we allowed the excess energy to discharge. As the energy was released and discharged from his chest and digestive systems, his symptoms were greatly relieved and eventually disappeared. The work we did gave his body time to complete the responses. As we discharged arousal related to the earth-quake, his stomach and intestines relaxed. Several weeks later he reported both the respiratory and stomach symptoms were almost completely gone.

The earthquake had ambushed Sam and he'd had to switch from a deep sleep state to a state of coping with intense danger in a split second. The more abrupt the shift we have to make to cope with threat, the more we tend to experience trapped excess energy and more intense trauma symptoms.

What Happens When Voltage Builds

When your body is overactivated, it grips inside and traps excess energy. It loses its capacity to discharge or let go. Remember how we compared your nervous system to an electrical system? When you can't discharge energy, the voltage builds. Symptoms tend to become more severe because it is an escalating process. Each time you attempt to reconnect with your body you may feel "zapped" again by the unresolved trauma. Your body has internalized the threat. Even when no actual danger is present, your body contin-ues to retrigger the threat response, causing trapped energy to build and symptoms to escalate.

There's a scene in the movie *Jurassic Park* that is completely incor-rect—and it has nothing to do with dinosaurs. A young boy is climb-ing an electric fence when the power is turned back on and he is thrown from the fence. In reality, when your body is exposed to too much voltage, you have to be peeled off the fence or the electricity has to be turned down! Your system constricts and you grip tightly, physically unable to let go.

Logjams

I like to equate the excess energy in your system to logjams. At first, excess energy stacks neatly, one event on the other, just as logs will move smoothly down a river side by side without interfering with one another. They easily slide under bridges or around narrow river bends. More events may cause energy to stack randomly, in the same way that logs may become disorganized, piling onto one another in a rough river current. At this stage, your body still can deal with the excess energy without overloading if it is given time and space to recover.

Energy Logjams—Levels of Activation in the Nervous System

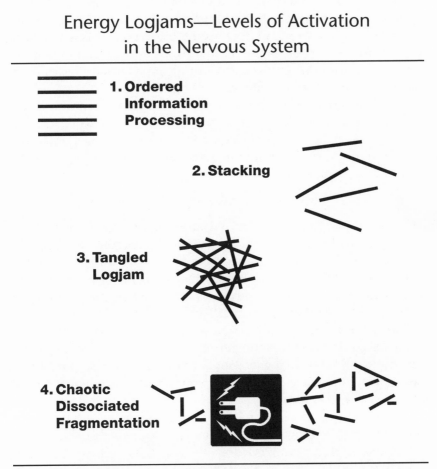

1. **Ordered Information Processing**

2. **Stacking**

3. **Tangled Logjam**

4. **Chaotic Dissociated Fragmentation**

As the system becomes overactivated, the excess energy piles up, chaotically creating a "logjam." Have you ever seen how logs can stack upon one another if one log blocks the others crosswise at a bridge abutment? Treatment at this stage deals with the tangled logjam energy like a child playing with pickup sticks, removing and discharging them one by one. I recall loggers in my hometown moving gingerly out onto the logjam, hooked poles in hand, freeing the logs one by one until the jam could clear. You don't have to get every log, or treat every symptom. You just need to deal with enough to get your system moving and resilient again.

When a client comes in and reports experiencing a headache, stomachache, tension, and nervousness all at once, this is a logjam. It can produce memory lapses, lack of concentration, and even more stress. Just explaining how some symptoms naturally result from overstimulation is often calming and reassuring.

The best way to overcome a logjam is by focusing on one symptom until it clears, then on the next. Unfortunately, when you are experiencing a logjam, you usually feel a sense of urgency and there is a tendency to speed up instead of slowing down.

Your Nervous System Just "Over-Ate"

Another way of thinking about logjamming or overload is to compare it to the digestive system. The autonomic nervous system works with life events much as the digestive system works with food. When everything is running smoothly, both systems take what they need and discard the rest. Your body does this automatically. You don't have to think about digesting breakfast or lunch. But think how you feel after a big meal such as Thanksgiving dinner. You have overloaded your digestive system. You may feel uncomfortable or even painfully full. You are groggy. Your digestion is no longer automatic. It becomes something that disturbs you. It takes a while to get food moving again comfortably.

If nervous system overstimulation continues, you can't deal with the stress, and it "blows up" or fragments. Going back to our image of loggers, when clearing one log at a time fails to dissipate a jam, sometimes dynamite is used to explode the logs and clear the channel. That works well for real logjams but when your nervous system deals with a major overload by fragmenting, you have what we have described as dissociation. This form of dissociation leaves you with highly charged pieces of memory separated by gaps in which you have no recollection of events. Treatment for this involves piecing together these highly charged fragments of memory and discharging each through resourcing, a technique you will learn in Chapter 6.

When you are fragmented you can't remember everyday information such as frequently used phone numbers. You may continually lose your car keys or your glasses. You may not feel your physical presence, or you may feel, as we commonly say, "beside yourself." Perhaps you feel disoriented in space, walking into door frames or furniture as a result.

The nervous system itself does not distinguish which trauma the voltage came from, so even if you don't have specific memories of your accident, discharging the "overwhelm." will reduce your activation. Once the excess energy is discharged, memory usually returns and the gaps decrease.

We want to help you avoid being blown from the fence or having to be peeled off. Instead, we want to teach you to reduce the voltage by gradually discharging it, much like gently turning down a dimmer switch. Together, we intentionally "chunk down" your experience into manageable pieces and give you resources to help you cope. Your body releases naturally and with ease.

Think of blowing up a balloon. If you blow it up too far—fill it with too much air—it bursts. Pieces become disconnected or "dissociated" from each other. If you fill it then let it go suddenly, it flies crazily around the room, much like a panic attack or outburst of rage. But if you let the air (energy) out slowly and gradually, the balloon gently goes limp. The energy is discharged without disruption.

We're helping you use the dimmer switch to bring the voltage down. As the voltage is reduced and activation is released, you'll immediately begin to feel better. This book is designed to guide you into sensing what your body wants or needs. Have faith in your body. It wants to heal and knows how to do it.

Expansion and Contraction

When you are traumatized, your body responds with contraction. This natural response is built into every organism, from a one-celled amoeba to a human being. Contraction makes us a smaller target.

Think about the tiny amoeba you studied in high school biology class. Remember how they shrivel up when prodded?

If you prick an amoeba with a pin, it pulls in its pseudopods, contracting into a circular shape. Then, gradually, it begins tentatively to reach out another pseudopod. It may pull back a bit, then reach out again. As you watch, more pseudopods will appear, and the amoeba moves out again to explore its world. It has recovered from the pinprick.

However, if you prick the amoeba again, giving it an additional trauma each time it stretches out a pseudopod, eventually it contracts and remains there. It ceases to explore. It is completely contracted. It has adapted to a narrow, avoidant reality.

Your body responds to trauma in the same way. Particularly if you have experienced extreme or multiple traumas, you're afraid to stick out a pseudopod! You are afraid to explore or engage in life. Everything is contracted—your relationships, your emotions, your senses, your body. Your life may become very narrow in an attempt to stay safe. The extreme form of this is agoraphobia or fear of open spaces.

Worse yet, you may have a tendency to repeat the trauma by unconsciously putting yourself in similar circumstances over and over. Called trauma re-enactment, this explains why people may have a series of rear-end accidents, or why battered women get out of one abusive relationship only to enter another.

I recall having lunch with an attorney who specializes in auto accident cases. He asked me to explain a strange phenomenon. "My files are full of records of clients who continue to have the same type of accident again and again," he said. I explained to him that people who have unresolved trauma may re-enact their accidents because they tend to overfocus on one aspect of their driving. For instance, if they have been hit from the right, they may overfocus on the right to confront the threat or block out right to avoid it. Until trauma victims can get themselves reoriented to their surroundings normally, they continue to be in danger of repeating the accident.

After trauma begins to be resolved, as you begin to reach out, there's expansion as the pent-up activation discharges. This may be followed by a contraction, as a counter-reaction to the expansion. It's not a linear process as you recover. You'll move slowly and begin to build on the expansion. It takes a lot of trust to put out that first pseudopod, but as your confidence and safety level grow, your nervous system will begin to restore itself to normal.

Developing a sense of safety in all stages of this work is crucial. If you start to feel unsafe, it means you are beginning to reactivate the trauma and need to begin resourcing, as we will discuss in the next chapter.

Key Points

- It is important to get an overall understanding of your symptoms

- When a person is overwhelmed by trauma, the overload causes energetic logjams

- Too much overload leads to fragmentation and dissociation

- In response to trauma many people react by narrowing their lives

6

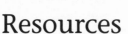

Resources

The approach to treating trauma presented in this book differs from other therapies or treatment approaches you might have tried. It is based on the idea that your body knows exactly what it needs for healing. It builds on your own natural resources, restoring your sense of self-worth and self-trust, while helping your nervous system regain balance and resiliency.

> Definition: A resource is any positive memory, person, place, action, or personal capacity that creates a soothing feeling in your body. We actively use these resources to help you reduce nervous system overactivation and stimulate a relaxation discharge response.

Resources are the positive experiences in our lives, past and present, including the people we know and love. Resources can also be parts of your body that feel good, even though other parts of your body may be in chronic pain from your accident. Our clients who have suffered from long-term debilitating chronic pain are always surprised that they can find some part of their body that actually still feels positive sensations.

Exercise: Experiencing a Resource

The goal of this exercise is to show you how thinking of a resource causes physical changes in your body.

Think of some place, time, or person that made you feel safe and relaxed. As you access that image, pay attention to what you feel in your body. As you focus on a resource, you may experience relaxation, perhaps with an increased sense of well-being. It should feel comforting and soothing. It is important that you pay attention to the details of the experience of well-being and how it feels inside your body. This is the beginning of creating an oasis of safety in the body. Take your time. Notice the variety of ways your body signals to you that it is relaxing. Notice any discharge of tension from your body.

Exercise: Learning How to Loop

This exercise helps you find those places in your body that feel comfortable and relaxed.

Sit quietly, both feet on the floor. Scan your body with your internal body awareness. See if you can find some place in you that feels soft, warm, and relaxed. Even if you have been in chronic pain, let your focus be on where you have positive feelings. Keep your awareness there. Notice how large the area may be that actually feels pleasant. Notice any sense of temperature, color, or movement.

After you get really acquainted with this spot, bring your awareness back into the edge of your pain or tension—but only for an instant! Then focus your attention back to where you feel good. Working from trauma activation to resource repetitively is one of the techniques we use to discharge activation. This process is called looping. Repeat this process several times, but only touch into the edge of the pain. Don't stay in it.

Many people report to their surprise that their pain begins to recede after this exercise. Notice that you are not trying to relax the part that is tight or in pain. That usually makes it worse. Pain is like a magnet; it is drawn to our consciousness like a tongue to a jagged tooth. Pain is often an indication of a logjam. By focusing our awareness on it, or even by trying to get it to relax, we are actually adding logs to the jam and making things worse.

When you're suffering from trauma symptoms, it may be difficult at first to find a resource. You're so focused on what's wrong that it's hard to focus on what's right. Pain overcomes all other interests or perspectives. Resources are always there. You wouldn't have lived this long without having access to certain resources, so if you have trouble finding one, you may just be disconnected from them at this moment. Just as your immune system automatically clicks in to heal when you cut your finger, your body resources kick in after you've experienced trauma. This book shows you how to access those resources to help your body heal.

What's Right with You, Anyway?

Traditional psychotherapy may tend to focus on what's gone wrong in your life. By contrast, this method will teach you how to work on what disturbs you, while at the same time remaining connected to what works (or has worked) well in your life as a resource. By learning to access your resources, you'll make it safe for your body to work through its biological responses to trauma.

It is important to focus on what is healthy in you. Often, patients come to me in such a state of discouragement and depression that they cannot see a way through their problems, especially if they have been involved in severe accidents. They see only the damage and the pain. I always reassure them that what I see is the health and the potential in them. I communicate to them that I am convinced that they have the strength to overcome their problems until, through treatment, they see that they can regain health.

It can really be helpful if you, your caregivers, and those around you remain focused on the conviction that healing is possible. Have you ever been with a friend or caregiver who is so focused on what's not working for you that it seems impossible to imagine that you will ever be better? Think how this feels, as opposed to being with someone who focuses on your capacities and strengths. You might want to explain to those around you that increasing focus on what's working gives you the resources you need to work on the symptoms that are holding you back from recovery.

Working together with the exercises in this book, we will establish an oasis of stability that you can return to when dealing with highly charged memories from the accident. Take a break whenever you feel overactivated by any of the exercises. You can practice switching back to your oasis or resources.

The goal is to recreate or enhance and build a sense of safety and support. This is not a "no pain, no gain" process. The breaks you take are as important as the work you do on the traumatic event.

Note: Only by switching back and forth from focusing on activation of the trauma to focusing on your resources can your nervous system gain the discharge and relaxation it needs. Regaining a sense of safety is paramount.

Exercise: Bringing Sensation Into the Body

Here's an exercise in resourcing. Let yourself feel the sensations in your body.

Think of a trip to Hawaii. Imagine yourself lying on the beach. Can you feel the sun on your body? Take a moment. Concentrate. Feel the warmth of the sun. What happens in your body when you feel yourself lying in the sun? Can you hear palms blowing in the breeze? Waves breaking on the shore? What happens in your body when you feel the warm sand beneath you, the warmth of the sun and a cool breeze? How are you affected? What sensation words fit what you are feeling? Give yourself several minutes to savor the sensation.

As you work, you'll constantly be moving back and forth between activation of the trauma and the discharge that results from accessing and feeling the resource in the body. This body responsiveness and potential for discharge of painful states are available to you all the time. You take them with you wherever you go.

Exercise: Resource into Sensation

Here's another short exercise to help you with experiencing your body more deeply.

Think of a person or a pet who is a resource to you—a spouse, parent, relative, friend, fictional character, or even your dog or cat. Close your eyes and concentrate on that resource. When you imagine their presence, how do you feel in your body? Responses are individual. Some people report sensations of expansion or relaxation, a deep sigh of relief (belly breathing) or warmth, or tingling in their fingertips. These sensations reflect that you are working directly with the parasympathetic nervous system (reptilian brain) and are discharging energy. Resourcing helps regulate the autonomic nervous system through discharging excess energy. Take your time with this. It is essential to give your body all the time it needs to access these resources.

Your Personal Resources

Here is a form to help you evaluate your personal resources. Include anything you can use to your advantage or that enhances your ability to deal effectively with problems or threats. Resources give you a feeling of warmth, safety, expansion, and comfort. They can be real or imaginary. For instance, your resources might include an imaginary place you would like to be, or an imaginary ally to help fight your battles. As you increase your menu of resources, your resiliency increases. Come back to your list from time to time, and see if you can add to your resources. On your list, include:

1. *Internal resources* are qualities, such as your intelligence, perseverance, ingenuity, confidence, competence, creativity, flexibility, sense of value or spirituality.

2. *External resources* are supports, such as friends and family members, favorite places, enjoyable sports, and positive memories.

3. *Missing resources* are those that currently feel unavailable or unused, such as lack of confidence, or lack of connection to friends.

Next is what a partially completed Personal Resource Inventory might look like:

INTERNAL RESOURCES:	EXTERNAL RESOURCES:	MISSING RESOURCES:
I know how to ask for what I need, I'm competent and quick-acting in high stress situations, I'm flexible and make changes relatively easily. I feel strong and healthy.	*My friend Patty is always there for me and I let her know when I need help. My boss understands my situation and lets me have a lighter schedule when needed. My husband rubs my back to help me calm down or go to sleep. I have a cabin in the mountains that I can escape to when I need to be alone. My dog, Serendipity, sleeps by the door and knows how to be protective. Whenever I think of my favorite uncle, Derrick, I feel safe and relaxed.*	*I can't connect to or communicate with my family about the accident. I have trouble getting help from my doctor about the insomnia I have had since the accident. I don't feel safe driving on highways or bridges any more. I feel a lot more isolated and miss feeling like being with my friends.*

You may want to make a simple list of resources. You may want to collect photos of your resources and keep them in a photo album. Do what works best for you.

Now fill out your own resource inventory sheet.

INTERNAL RESOURCES:	EXTERNAL RESOURCES:	MISSING RESOURCES:

Personal Resource Inventory
to Enhance Resiliency

Take a look at your list. You may see that your resources are clustered in certain areas, while other areas may seem less full. For instance, you may have many resources in the sports or outdoors area, but none involving people. It's a good way to assess your areas of strength and guide you to areas where you might need to expend more effort to find resources in them. You can never have too many resources, internal or external.

Time Line

Here's another chart which may help to show you how you have already been using resources to help throughout your life. First, think of an overwhelming event. Mark it in at the age when it happened to you. Then opposite the event, think of resources that were available to you at the time. We've filled in some examples for you.

OVERWHELMING EVENT	AGE	RESOURCES
	60	
	55	
	50	
Divorce	45	Friends, support
	40	
	35	
Auto accident	30	Good medical care, supportive husband, dedication to my rehab program
	25	
	20	
Father Died	15	Church, best friend, dog, playing soccer
	10	
	5	
	Birth	

Now fill out your own time line.

OVERWHELMING EVENT	AGE	RESOURCES

You can never have too many resources. It is a good idea to always be on the lookout for ways to expand your available resources. Sometimes that process requires noting an area where resources seem insufficient and working specifically on what gets in the way of accessing those resources. The more resources you have in your life, the more resiliency you will have in dealing with life's challenges. Often it is helpful to ask a friend to explore with you which of your resources seem intact and are actively working for you and which ones you might have difficulty tapping into.

Competent Protectors

The younger you are when a traumatic event occurs, the more you need the presence of a protective ally as a resource. Children absolutely need competent, protective adults in their lives. So often survivors of childhood abuse have rarely or never known protection. This is an example of a missing resource that has severe implications. As children and then as adults, these people may have the feeling that there is no safe haven for them.

If you're not listing any people as resources—often the loss of trust results in the survivor's reluctance to rely on other people— consider whether there might be someone trustworthy enough to add as a resource. It doesn't have to be a living person or even a real one at first. People have varying capacities and areas in which they can help or support us.

Don

Don's trauma arose from childhood abuse, as well as memories of his parents constantly fighting. He identified one key resource. His Aunt Sadie tried her best to protect him from his abusive parents. When he mentioned her, I suggested he remember her face and experience what happens in his body when he did that. As he envisioned her kind face and felt her loving presence, he said he felt calmed and protected. I asked him how he experienced the sense of protection in his body. Don reported feeling softness and warmth begin to spread out through his torso and noticed that his chronically tight shoulders gradually relaxed. He was actually learning what safety and protection felt like physically. The significant point here is that we were able to use his real feelings for his aunt to begin to build a sense of safety for him in the present that he could access internally.

Some people use their religious faith as a resource, actively calling on Jesus Christ, the Buddha, or other religious figures. Once a protective ally is re-established, the client usually feels the desire and possibility for self-protection. In everyday life we need to know how to ask for support from others as well as how to protect ourselves when needed.

Margaret

Margaret found that the inventory of resources that she developed to help her nervous system discharge were insufficient when she began working toward the moment of impact. She became overwhelmed.

She was a deeply religious person and found that only the image of Jesus in the car with her helped her manage her extreme activation and the trauma related to the impact. Using Jesus as her protective ally allowed her to work slowly through the most highly traumatizing moments of her accident.

Other clients have mentally brought a loving grandparent or their spouse to help them deal with the most difficult moments of their accident. The important thing to remember with any resource is that it is valid if it has a soothing effect on a person's nervous system. That is why it is so important that these images, memories, etc., come from your own experience or imagination, not as a suggestion from a therapist. Events of the accident or trauma can cause you to lose resources, as in the case of one of my clients, Natalie.

Natalie

Natalie came to me to work on a phobic reaction to dogs that she simply couldn't understand. As we worked, Natalie slowly began to recall a traumatic event from her youth. At the age of nine, she was brutally attacked by two strange men on the way to a soccer game. Afterward, she had total amnesia about the event. Because it was so terrible and unmanageable to her as a young girl, the event was completely blocked from her memory.

She knew something terrible had happened, but couldn't remember what. Because she wasn't sure who or what had harmed her, she pulled away from friends and family. She didn't know who she could trust. Because she felt such anxiety around her family, especially her father, she became suspicious that he may have hurt her. As a result, they were lost as resources for her.

Working through the incident, all Natalie could remember at first was the sight of trees and sky above her during the attack. Then she remembered hearing the sound of barking dogs that were fenced in nearby. When we are in serious danger, our reptilian brain takes a "snapshot" of the circumstances. This snapshot may include many aspects of the situation such as sounds, sights, smells, time of day, the weather, or colors that are associated with the trauma. Any of these may then become fearful triggers later on. A well-known example of that phenomenon is a Vietnam veteran reacting to the sound of a traffic helicopter by flashing back to Vietnam.

Even though the phobia Natalie wanted to treat was related to barking dogs, the real issue was related to the attackers. As we gradually dealt with the assault, her fears became appropriately associated with the two men and their terrible actions. She was able to work through the assault bit by bit and eventually could handle the experience and felt freer from its negative impact.

During treatment, I suggested that the dogs might have been trying to protect her, not harm her. She felt deep inside that that was true for her. Her fear of dogs disappeared. In fact, she eventually began to have very positive feelings toward dogs as protectors.

As treatment progressed, and her feelings of helplessness diminished, Natalie was able to access her natural feeling of self-defense. She was able to imagine herself pushing away the assailants. She could feel her body organize the muscles in her back and shoulders and feel the necessary strength inside her to push them away. She could feel the adult power that was available to her now coming to help the overwhelmed and overpowered child from years earlier. This is only one example of how completing a successful action of self-defense was very empowering to Natalie. As she was able to regain more and more of a sense of power and strength, the sense of previous weakness and overwhelming helplessness became *less and less. These same techniques can help you overcome the feelings of powerlessness you may have experienced during your auto accident.*

Gradually, as her memories returned, Natalie realized her family was not involved in the attack and they became resources for her as she reconnected with them.

Giving Yourself Time

The one resource that is almost always missing in auto accident trauma is time.

Your accident most likely happened so quickly that your body did not have time to react. Giving yourself time is very reassuring to the reptilian brain. Do not rush yourself through the exercises or memories.

Exercise: Freeze Frame

This exercise shows you how adding more time to your experience can change your sensations.

Perhaps you are having a repetitive image of the car from your accident coming toward you. Now imagine that the car stops moving toward you at a safe distance away—whatever that distance might be for you. This technique is called freeze-frame.

It might be a few feet or a few miles, but it needs to be close enough that you begin to feel the car as a threat. What happens in your body when you see the car from a safe distance and freeze frame it there so it can't move? Giving yourself distance from the threat helps you remain connected to your body. Focusing on the threat then makes some clients feel an urge to run—a flight response. Others feel angry—a fight response. What happens in your body when you have these feelings? You may feel hot, or flushed. You may panic, or you may have an impulse or need for physical action. Find out what your body wants to do. Then imagine your body preparing itself to fight or flee. Pay close attention to how that feels in your body. Complete the visualization slowly while you continue to sense your body. If this exercise brings relief, notice how you experience that sense of relief physically.

Your own body is your most potent resource. There are activation symptom areas and areas where you feel comfortable. You need to become aware of both. Your activation area may be an area in which you have no sensation at all—perhaps a sense of feeling cut off from your legs. A scary experience can disconnect us from our feelings of self. As the activation dissipates, your sense of self will return, and all the parts will be there. Conduct a body scan from time to time and see how your self-awareness increases.

Exercise: Contact and Grounding

The goal of this exercise is to focus on your body and to add the resource of grounding.

Sit in a comfortable chair. Think about where your body is in contact with the chair. How does it feel? How does your chest feel? Do you feel any sensations in your stomach? What about your arms? Are they heavy? Tingling? Take as much time as you need to examine your sensations.

Can you feel both your legs? If not, press your feet against the floor. Does this change your awareness of your legs? What sensations do they feel? Now imagine that your legs could have anything they want. What would help them feel more connected to your body? Think back to a part of your body that feels comfortable. Feel that sensation. Now return to your numb area. Is there anything that would make it feel more comfortable?

As you work through the exercise, you may be aware of a feeling of warmth or expansion. This is a sign the energy is discharging. You may feel trembling or shaking. Remember the dog? Your body is releasing trapped energy just as the dog's body did after a near miss. This is a good sign. It shows you your body knows how to restore itself when given the chance.

Remember, it's not that you can't handle normal stress or activation. Your problem is that your nervous system has been subjected to overwhelming events—too much, too fast, too soon. Resources help you discharge excess energy trapped in your body, allowing you to return to your natural state of resiliency where you can handle everyday stresses again without feeling overwhelmed.

Using Your Resource Inventory

Use your resources whenever you feel threatened or overwhelmed. Create a resource inventory for yourself. Don't try to work on your trauma until you have a resource inventory. Once you feel the body's ability to find just the right resource, it's incredibly confidence-building. Learning to create resources is an important life skill that not only helps relieve the trauma of the accident, but also prepares you for future life challenges.

Resource Suggestions from Clients

One client listed all the good things that happened to her on pieces of paper and put them in a cookie jar. Whenever she felt bad, she pulled out resources and read them until she felt better. Another used a photo album with pictures of people and places that were her resources. As she looked through the album, she would feel the sensations evoked by each resource. Another client is at work on a "resource room," where everything from the comfortable chair to the pictures on the walls represent resources to her.

Useful Metaphors

Many clients find water to be a useful resource or metaphor for safe driving. They often find water images, such as swimming, sailing, or visualizing themselves at the seashore, to be particularly helpful. The flow of water seems to replicate the flow of energy that supports a sense of well-being.

Jolene

Jolene had a lot of trouble focusing on her driving after her rear-end accident. She was too conscious of what was happening behind her. Driving was difficult, especially since she couldn't see herself being in control of the car. She wanted to be in the back seat with someone else in control. She couldn't imagine ever enjoying driving again.

Jolene grew up sailing, and found it secure and soothing. We had her use sailing imagery as a resource. She easily could envision herself at the helm of the boat, controlling its movement with the tiller. As she used the imagery, she began to connect the flow of water around the boat with the normal flow of traffic. She visualized cars as a school of fish, all turning automatically in response to changes in the roadway. Instead of seeing each car around her as an individual hostile barrier, Jolene began to see the symmetry and orchestration of normal traffic flow. As her resources increased, she was able to see other drivers as friendly and skillful, rather than as neglectful and reckless. This is an example of moving from defensive orienting to normal exploratory orienting.

Resisting Resources

As you begin work, you may find it difficult to access resources. Some people push their resources away. You may be so avoidant that you simply don't want to talk about your trauma. You just want the accident not to have happened. Wanting to shut down is a common response. For other people, relaxation may actually feel dangerous— as if letting your guard down invites attack or threat.

In this case we work with clients to separate out this fear that has become associated with the relaxation response.

Resourced and Ready!

Go back to your resource inventory on page 69 and see if you can fill the sheet now.

Exercise: Starting the Work

The goal of this exercise is to begin gaining resiliency.

Think of a time when you've felt safe. Concentrate on these feelings. Where were you? Who was with you? How did that feel in your body? Were you relaxed? How was your breathing?

Think of the point in the accident when you knew something was wrong. What happened in your body at that moment? What would have made you feel safer? Was there someone you thought of when you thought of safety? How would having that person with you make you feel? What might they have said to you? What would they have done? What happens in your body when you imagine their presence?

Henry

Henry's car slid on the ice and hit a tree. He suffered a head injury so serious that he had to quit his job. Henry was extremely resistant to working on the accident. He simply didn't want to discuss it.

Many psychotherapists refer to this avoidant attitude as "the client's resistance." We disagree with this. It places blame. We feel that there is always a door to resiliency and urge you not to give up in finding yours.

With Henry, the key was his love of playing the cello. He became very anxious before a performance. Together, we began to work on that issue and Henry began to visualize himself performing with confidence. He could feel grounded in his body and the joy of playing the music as he began to understand how resourcing works. Once he started to trust the technique, it opened the door to working on his accident trauma symptoms.

Key Points

• Your body knows what it needs to heal

• Everyone has his or her own set of resources

• Learning to work with these resources can help you heal

• Exercises in this chapter help you access your resources on a sensation level, rather than a mental level

• Slowing down is a resource

• Reconnecting to your body experience is a resource

7

$\backsim$

Restoring Resiliency

By nature, humans are quite resilient. We have the ability to overcome great obstacles and bounce back. Only when our systems are totally overwhelmed by traumatic events do we lose this natural resiliency.

It's important to stop and take stock of the various resources in your life to understand your own resiliency factors.

Your Personal Resiliency Quotient

Some people have more natural resiliency than others. There are many variables. Genetics seems to play a role. Some people simply have stronger immune systems and heal from physical or emotional injuries more quickly. Your resiliency may be undermined by multiple traumas, or bolstered by good support systems. When your healing begins, you will find that the process tends to escalate. The more resources you discover and resiliency you build, the faster healing occurs.

Resiliency is contagious too. Therapists we have trained find that when they use resiliency as a key element in treatment, they are far less drained at the end of the day. As our clients gain resiliency, we are inspired and become more resilient as well.

The Heller Resiliency Scan

The questions listed in the Heller Resiliency Scan are suggestions to help you identify additional resources in several suggested areas of your life.

Work Resiliency

What type of work are you doing now?

_____

_____

What do you like about your work?

_____

_____

_____

_____

What kind of relationships do you have with the people you work with/for?

_____

_____

_____

_____

What are your career goals/dreams?

_____

_____

_____

_____

Does your current position fit with your career goals/dreams?

_____

_____

If not, how might you find a more satisfying career?

_____

_____

_____

Relationship Resiliency

Partners

Are you currently in a fulfilling intimate partnership?

_____

What do you like about your relationship?

_____

_____

_____

If you are not in an intimate relationship, do you want one or would you prefer to be alone?

_____

_____

Describe your relationship with your partner.

_____

_____

_____

How do you and your partner resolve conflicts?

_____

_____

_____

_____

Do you feel you both have good communication skills?

_____

How do you feel about commitment?

_____

_____

_____

What kind of resources for support do you and your partner have outside of the relationship?

_____

_____

_____

How might you both expand your range of resources together?

_____

_____

_____

Individually?

_____

_____

_____

Family

What kind of relationship do you have with your family?

_____

_____

_____

How does your family deal with conflict?

_____

_____

_____

In what areas does the family experience difficulties?

_____

_____

_____

What kind of support system does the family have within it and outside of it?

_____

_____

_____

How might the family's resource base be enhanced?

_____

_____

_____

Parenting

If you have children, describe yourself as a parent.

_____

_____

_____

What resources can you, your child, or the family draw on for aid when needed?

_____

_____

_____

In what ways can the support available be broadened?

_____

_____

_____

_____

Social Support System

What type of relationships do you have with friends?

_____

_____

What do you like about your relationships with your friends?

_____

_____

What do you usually base friendship on? (i.e., activities, emotional support, similarities.)

_____

_____

_____

Are your friendships generally satisfying?

_____

_____

Do you enjoy a sense of belonging and connectedness?

_____

_____

Life Purpose, Path, and Passion

Do you have a dream or specific path you are pursuing?

_____

If not, do you know when you disconnected from your dream?

_____

_____

What personal goals do you feel enthusiastic about?

_____

_____

What professional goals inspire you?

_____

_____

Do you have professional mentors? How can they help you?

_____

_____

_____

What areas of your life inspire passion, enthusiasm, and meaning?

_____

_____

_____

What might help you increase the possibility of fulfilling these goals?

_____

_____

_____

Coping Skills and Strategies

How do you deal with problems that arise in your life?

_____

_____

_____

What are your positive ways to self soothe? (massage or exercise versus drinking alcohol or over-eating, for example)

_____

_____

How do you recover from a disruptive or disturbing event?

_____

_____

Who in your support system do you most rely on?

_____

_____

Health and Fitness

How would you describe your level of health and vitality?

_____

_____

_____

How would you describe your nutrition habits?

_____

_____

_____

What kind of exercise do you enjoy?

_____

_____

_____

How many hours of sleep do you get each night?

_____

_____

What do you do when you are not feeling well?

_____

_____

_____

Do you have a good health care support system?

_____

_____

Interests and Activities

Do you have a variety of interests and hobbies, such as reading, gardening, dancing, collections, cooking, riding, or enjoying pets?

_____

_____

_____

How can you expand your creative interests and choices?

_____

_____

_____

Spiritual Growth

What is your spiritual focus or religious orientation?

_____

_____

How do you feel about your orientation/focus?

_____

_____

_____

Do you feel connected to something greater than yourself?

_____

_____

How does your belief affect your healing process?

_____

_____

_____

_____

Oasis of Safety

Creating an Oasis

Before we begin working on your accident, we are going to help you create an oasis, a safe place for you to be. We began this work in Chapter 6 and will continue it here. You must have solid ground to work from before you step off into the emotional and physical quicksand of your accident.

An oasis is a collection of resources that creates a feeling of a solid foundation. As we work together on the events of the accident, you'll be adding additional resources and thinking of other positive things that you did or know of or might have done. I'll help you create an oasis at each end of your experience—your resources before and after the accident—as we add more resources and dissipate the activation. You will work on building a bridge of resources to span the event.

One of the greatest resources you have is the present. *You already accomplished the most important part of the work—you survived.* Now we need to clear up any residual problems you're having from the accident. We can't change the facts of what happened, but we can greatly affect the way the event is impacting you now.

Exercise: It's Not Over 'Til It's Over

The goal of this exercise is to help your reptilian brain realize that you survived. Our neocortex may know that, but if the reptilian brain hasn't relaxed yet, it is still triggered for danger.

Try saying these phrases and notice how you feel in your body:

"I survived."
"I made it."
"I'm alive"
"What I did worked"
"I'm here"
"It's over"

As you say each phrase aloud, focus on your body. How does it feel? What's happening? How does your chest feel? Your breathing? Do you notice a tightness anywhere? As it loosens, what do you notice happening in your body? If your body could dissipate that energy, how might it like to do that?

As you heal, it's common to feel a sense of aliveness, enthusiasm, or increased energy as you work through this exercise. Give yourself time to experience each sensation. People react in a variety of ways to saying these statements aloud and your reaction can give an indication of whether or not your body actually registers that the threat has passed and that you are now really out of danger.

Often at the beginning of treatment our clients may report feeling nothing or numbness in response to these statements as if they didn't apply to them. They feel that their survival isn't real even though cognitively they know they did in fact survive.

As treatment progresses and a person becomes more connected to the impact of what happened to them, they may feel intense grief or sadness. Eventually a person may feel tremendous relief in the felt realization of their survival. As the trauma resolves and healing has been completed a person may report feeling a sense of accomplishment, mastery or exhilaration. "I made it and I'm alive" then becomes joyous and real.

Repeating these phrases aloud at different intervals during recovery is diagnostic and can give you feedback on your progress.

That Disconnected Feeling

People generally feel a sense of well-being when they connect to their sense of aliveness. So what if you don't feel a sense of relief when you say, "I'm alive?" This is a strong signal that you're still feeling very disconnected. Remember, it's perfectly natural to feel disconnected after a frightening experience. Go back to Chapter 4 and repeat the exercises to help you connect to your body. Once the reptilian brain "clicks on" again to the knowledge that you are alive, you will experience a tremendous sense of relief.

> What You Need To Know: Surviving is biological success.
> It doesn't matter how you did it.

Trauma Time Zones

Our body/mind operates in present tense. You may still feel like the accident just happened even though it is months or years in the past. You are still reacting as if the trauma is here. You may even experience "flash forwards" or futurized memory. Some of my clients tell me they visualize an accident occurring again as they approach an intersection—a signal that their nervous system is still stuck in the "scanning to locate threat" mode. As you resolve the trauma, you will feel the experience moving back into its proper time—the past. You have an important resource. You DID survive. The body needs to be reminded.

It's important that you feel you have a safe place to be before you proceed to work on the accident itself. If you still don't feel safe, take some time to think about other times in life when you felt safe. This helps you build an association with safety and create a foundation for the next exercises.

Exercise: Establishing a Sense of Safety

The goal of this exercise is to help your body remember how safety feels.

When was the first time you felt safe after the accident? (Your answer may be that you don't feel safe yet. That's okay. These exercises will help you re-establish safety.) If you haven't felt safe since the accident, remember when you last felt safe before the accident. Where were you? Who was with you? What do you feel in your body when you remember that safe time?

What would make you feel safe now? Which people in your life make you feel protected or safe? What happens in your body when you think of these people?

If you don't have a real person in your life who makes you feel safe and protected, imagine a protective ally. What would he or she be like? Would he or she know what you need without your telling them? How might he or she help you feel safe? What would you want a competent protector to do? What happens in your body when you imagine someone acting protective toward you?

Do you have a place that makes you feel safe? One of my clients feels safe when she is in her bedroom with her dog. Another likes to be in the mountains or at the beach. Where is your safe place? Imagine that you are there. What happens in your body when you think of your safe place? Remember, it doesn't matter if these images seem silly or unrealistic. If they trigger a relaxation response, they are exactly what is needed.

What If I Can't Do This?

Just like accessing the reptilian brain, resourcing can take a little practice to feel comfortable. At first, you'll probably deal in factual resources—your family, your personal skills, a favorite possession, safe locations, and positive memories. As you visualize what might have been, you'll be surprised at how your reptilian brain begins to provide "what if" scenarios that get progressively more fanciful, yet help release the excess energy locked in your nervous system.

Evelyn

Evelyn, an international tax attorney, had a great deal of difficulty iden-tifying resources after her accident. In her first sessions, she could deal only with facts, so I used factual resources to help her—reassurances that she had survived, images of her husband as a comforting person, and how she feels around him.

As she worked more deeply into the details of the accident, she gradually began to visualize imaginary resources. By the end of several sessions, she was coping with her memory of the oncoming car by visualizing her-self bearing down on it in a huge semi-truck, pushing it out of her way. Imagining herself large, powerful, and in control counteracted her feel-ings of being small and helpless at the time of the accident. These images helped her body discharge the powerlessness and "overwhelm" that she had experienced since the accident.

Of course we can't change what actually happened. Resourcing helps our body restore itself to balance by allowing it to start moving out of the freeze response it has felt since the accident.

Key Points

- Humans are naturally resilient—some more than others

- The Resiliency Scan helps you establish your personal resiliency level

- An "oasis" gives you a feeling of safety and a foundation from which to work

- Feeling your reaction to saying phrases like "I'm alive" lets you know where you are in the healing process

- Never start working on difficult material without first establish-ing a felt experience of an oasis

- Trauma needs to move into the past where it belongs

8

~

Constructing Corrective Experiences

I've found several techniques helpful in healing trauma. One that works very well for most people is constructing alternatives to the accident. Peter Levine states in *Waking the Tiger*, "We must realize that it is neither necessary nor possible to change past events. . . . We have only to heal our present symptoms and proceed."

The goal of using a corrective experience is not to change your memory of what happened, but to let your mind and body play out alternative scenarios, imagining events the way you would have liked them to unfold. This helps create a competing physiological experience in your body, creating another option for your body that helps discharge trapped energy.

Exercise: Corrective Experience

The goal of this exercise is to orient you to including fantasy in your resources.

Think of the first moment that you realized the accident was happening. If you could have changed anything about that moment, what would it be? For example, if you had sped up and successfully avoided the collision, what kind of difference would you feel in your body?

Some of my clients find it comforting to visualize the oncoming car from an imaginary distance of several blocks (or even miles!) giving them the time to absorb the event that they did not have at the time of the accident. Others imagine themselves encased in foam rubber or pillows, so the impact is reduced. You might envision the impact under water, where the cars easily float apart. Some of my clients visualize themselves and the other driver in a bumper car game at the fair, where choice is available and the intention is to hit one another and bounce away. If you are able to visualize such an option, how does it feel in your body? Do you feel a sense of expansion or relaxation?

What if you could have had someone special (real or imaginary) there with you? How would the accident have been different? What might they have done? How do you feel when you think about what they might have done to help? One of Larry's patients felt the presence of God with her during the accident. Focusing on that experience and letting the impact of that particular resource filter through her nervous system made her healing go much more quickly.

This exercise may help you feel more comfortable with fantasizing resources. Trust your body to think of things that would have felt comforting or protective. Don't restrict yourself to facts. Let your imagination take over. You may surprise yourself with your own creativity!

Here's an example of how I used resources with one client to relieve his symptoms. Usually all your body remembers after an accident is the trauma, the fear, and the powerlessness. Using resources, I try to help my clients create an alternate physical sense or competing physiological experience.

David Rippe

As David made a left turn onto a two-lane highway, a drunk driver attempted to pass him at 80 miles per hour. His car was struck broadside. His first "Oh, no" moment was when he heard the impact and the sound of shattering glass. After the accident, any similar sounds reactivated his trauma responses. If someone dropped a glass, the shattering sound caused him to go into a state of high activation.

Because his strongest memory was the sound—in fact, at first David couldn't remember the rest of the accident—we started there. I had him focus on sounds he liked, such as wind in the trees or the song of a meadow lark, and asked him to assess what happened in his body when he heard those sounds. I asked him to imagine that he had heard those sounds during the accident. Invariably, he experienced a relaxation response that helped discharge energy. We would then shift to his memory of hearing glass shatter, and again I would have him describe what happened in his body. After we shifted back and forth three or four times, in a process we call looping, David could remember hearing glass shatter without having any reaction in his body. At that point we were ready to work on the next piece he remembered from the accident. Sometimes symptoms like these can take longer than three or four times, but often the speed with which some symptoms can be alleviated is astonishing.

Corrective experiences don't change what really happened, but they can create a bodily sense of what might have happened. They open you to other possibilities, like having a competing voice in your head; another internal experience grounded in your body to draw on. As my clients and I use this reworking of the events, we're imagining what might have happened in an ideal world. We experiment with how that might have made things different for them. Obviously, since they have had a serious accident, theirs is not an ideal world; nevertheless, playing out what a different scenario would feel like gives many clients a great deal of relief and reassurance and helps them begin shifting from trauma to healing.

> Remember: Trauma is in the nervous system. Whatever helps the nervous system move from frozenness and overwhelm back to a sense of flow is healing.

Sometimes you get stuck in traumatic memories. Perhaps you can't get the image of wreckage out of your mind. Sometimes an abrupt shift in focus can be helpful. When you feel stuck in a traumatic image, without worrying about the logic of it, imagine an opposite image. This corrective technique almost always helps you access a resource. Be aware of what happens in your body when you see the positive image.

One client, Maggie, kept seeing an activating image of the bright surgery lights during an operation she experienced after her accident. When asked to imagine an opposite, she saw soft candlelight. As she focused on the candlelight her body relaxed. When she revisited the surgery lights, they had become softer and less frightening.

Another client, Ted, felt frozen, like an empty mummy on an iceberg—an image significant of deep shock. When imagining the opposite—for him a pond with gentle ripples on a summer day—he began to feel gradually warmer and eventually fuller. This image helped him slowly move out of shock.

Exercise: Using the Power of Opposites

If you feel stuck in a particular difficult state of feeling such as a dark heaviness, depression, tightness, or constriction somewhere in your body, focus on this state. Then, without thinking about it, imagine what the opposite might be. The opposite you find may be unexpected, like an image of cotton candy for instance. It often initiates being in contact with a resource state that can help you move through the difficult state.

Part 1: What is the traumatic image or state that recurs for you?

_____

_____

_____

What is the opposite?

_____

_____

What do you feel in your body when you imagine the opposite?

_____

_____

Part 2: Now touch in to the original negative state or image. Do you feel the arousal connected to it increase or decrease? Go back to the opposite when you feel ready and notice how your body feels this time.

"Antidote" Resources

Corrective experience techniques can help you replace or restore missing resources. Perhaps you have a good resource system now, but did not at the time of the accident. Bring your present resources back to the past. What would the people who are your resources now have said to you at the time of the accident? What would they have done for you? Knowing what you know now, what might you say to the traumatized part of you?

The Rebound Effect

When you do corrective experiencing, there may be a "rebound" effect. Once you obtain resources, there may be a dual reality of relief and despair. Initially, you may experience relief, followed immediately by painful emotional reactions such as anger, hurt, or disappointment at being reminded of the suffering you've been experiencing. As you continue to work, this feeling will begin to heal. Resolution occurs and the pain can be left behind. You will be ready to move ahead.

Transformation

Trauma is a natural, normal part of life. Your body/mind is designed to heal intense or extreme experiences. Symptoms are not the actual problem—they signal the place where you need to begin your work, the areas of activation in your body where energy is trapped and the emotional triggers that need to be neutralized.

Definition: Transformation is a restoration of the losses
and a healing of the after-effects of trauma.

Once you have learned to release the trapped energy that results from interruption of the natural fight-or-flight instinct, you will feel:

• A new capability, a sense of "I can"

• A sense of control and safety

- Awareness of a wide range of choices and options

- Movement toward a sense of empowerment

- Awareness of your survival and an active choice toward life

- Ability to rest and relax

- Restoration of fluidity and flow

- A sense of completion and integration

Why Me?

Many trauma survivors repeat over and over, "Why me? Why did this happen?" These are the most difficult questions they must deal with. Perhaps the need to ask why comes from an instinctive need to avoid repeating the behavior that we believe got us into trouble, or the question may reflect a need to adapt by learning to locate danger. Trauma happens. We are physical beings on a physical planet and therefore physically vulnerable. We have bodies, minds, spirits, and emotions that can be wounded. We all have misfortune to deal with and to recover from. In any event, until you are able to move beyond "why me?" and accept that this accident has happened— regardless of the often unanswerable *why*—you may be unable to move on to successful treatment. All your energies will be focused on solving this often impossible riddle, when what you need is to begin healing. Healing can happen now as you learn to focus on your resources through the exercises in this book.

The same is true of feelings of blame. You can get locked into blaming yourself or another person involved in the accident and be so angry that you can't move forward. Blame is a normal response that humans have after trauma. It is often a way we try to manage our feelings of helplessness. Similar to getting stuck with "why me?", blaming ourselves or others keeps us from moving ahead with our healing. Sometimes blaming is a way to channel unresolved energy from a fight-or-flight response. In Chapter 6 we discussed a more useful way of channeling that energy. Be clear. I am not saying, "just get over it." I realize that when someone has caused you or a loved one a great deal of pain, that wound itself may take a great length of time to heal.

Key Points

- Trauma is held in the body in the form of energetic overload and negative images

- Corrective images and "antidote" resources must come from a person's own experience

- Alternative, corrective images—even fanciful—facilitate discharge and release and give your body access to a different physiological possibility

- Coming to terms with blocks to healing—"why me?", blame, and the need for revenge

9

⤳

Your Accident

Remember: If you become stressed at any time, go back and do some
of the resiliency exercises. Do not attempt to work through this
material too quickly.

Hopefully, you understand from earlier chapters what has happened
to your nervous system and why you are having some of the symptoms that disturb you. Now you know that these symptoms are a
common result of the autonomic nervous system's thwarted response
to danger. The symptoms arising from nervous system trauma aren't
permanent. Your body can heal them.

Chapter 6 showed you how to create a personal inventory of
resources and use exercises to calm yourself and discharge energy.
You have learned how to get in touch with your reptilian brain and
how to let your body tell you what it needs in order to heal.

Evaluating Your Post-Accident Symptoms

Several things may be happening to you that are direct results of
your accident:

- You may not feel safe when you are driving. Can you identify specific circumstances that trigger fear, rage, or a feeling of hyperarousal? Remember the linking action of your brain. It may surprise

you to realize that you are angry or fearful every time you see a car of the same make or color that hit you.

- You may feel disoriented while driving. You may miss exits, fail to be aware of intersections, or get lost more often.

- You may experience flashbacks, including sounds, intrusive imagery, trauma-related dreams, panic or anxiety attacks. You may visualize other cars hitting you, or hear the loud, crashing sound of the impact.

- You may visualize the accident happening again in the future. Maybe each time you approach an intersection, you envision cars running the light. When you brake on the freeway, you may picture someone hitting you from behind. This usually represents a disruption in time. Your awareness is trapped in that moment before the accident occurred and sees it about to happen. When you deactivate the charge of the accident, it will retreat into the past where it belongs. Until your perception of the accident returns to the past, you may be in danger of having the same or similar accident again. It is essential for your driving safety that you work through this phase.

- You may feel a lack of confidence in your own driving, or that of others.

- You may realize you have underdeveloped or underused driving skills that you need to enhance or restore. Could the accident have been prevented if you had used your horn? Practice finding your horn quickly. Could glare have been reduced by having a cleaner windshield?

- You may feel "not quite yourself" or fragmented.

Post-Accident Care

Again, events after the accident can influence your experience.

- Did you rest after the accident? Where? Could you really rest? Can you rest now? Do you feel hyper-vigilant and overcautious? Doing the exercises in this book should help restore your capacity to rest.

- Are you satisfied with your current caregivers? Do you need to coordinate treatment between several caregivers?

- Are you taking medications?

Use the body map to draw current injuries and pain patterns, as well as previous injuries. (For instance, seat-belt pressure may trigger pain from a previous abdominal incision.) What injuries did you receive during the accident?

Body Map

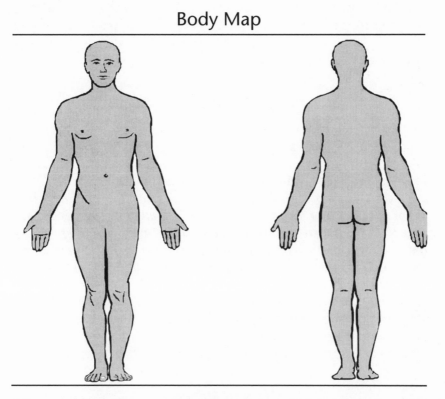

What outcomes do you want from treatment? Have the treatments you've received been inadequate or ineffective? Have you felt blamed for your symptoms?

Don't Tell it All

It's time for us to begin work on your accident. A very important part of the technique is that you will NOT go through details of the entire accident chronologically. We don't want you to tell your story from start to finish. Yes, the entire story is important, and eventually we will work on everything you experienced. But it is crucial that you deal with your accident piece by piece.

Why? Because retelling the accident from start to finish—as we all tend to do after such a traumatic experience—can retrigger the feelings you experienced and activate you physically into "over-whelm." It may intensify your trauma, not defuse it. I found that retelling the story of my accident made me feel worse. After you complete your work, you will be able to talk about the accident without retriggering your trauma. Use the following process.

Exercise: Safety After the Accident

First, to help establish a sense of safety, try to determine the moment you first felt safe after the accident. If you can, try to recall that first moment of even partial safety, such as the moment your husband arrived at the emergency room, or turning around to see that your child was unhurt, or even when a caring paramedic arrived on the scene. Once you have that memory, notice how the memory impacts you on a physical level. Take time to enjoy the sense of safety that arises in your body. After you are able to access a feeling of safety after the accident, we will process what happened before the accident. At each stage, we will loop back and forth between the events of the accident and your various resources, so that you are not overwhelmed by the memories. If you have not felt safe at all since the accident, we will be working with you in a different way. We will invite you to remember a time or circumstance where you felt safe in your life prior to the accident, then explore how that memory affects your body.

David Rippe

Here is what David told me about his first feelings of safety after the accident.

The truck that hit him shoved his car sideways 183 feet. David said he experienced relief when he felt his car finally stop in a ditch. Since the accident happened quite near his home, his family was available to him immediately.

We spent time helping David "deepen" his experience of grounding, and through visualization, gave his body plenty of time to relax and take in what had happened, instead of rushing out of the car as he did originally.

When you are able to deal with events before and after the accident without feeling overwhelmed, we'll work with healing some of your symptoms, working back and forth from activation to resource to release the energy. Remember what I did with David to defuse his reaction to the thought or actuality of the sound of breaking glass by using pleasant sounds as resources? We won't work with the actual moment of impact, the most activating moment of the accident, until you have discharged enough activation to be able to deal with the stress.

We call this working the "periphery of the accident." By working through the details from before the impact to after the impact, we will help you gradually loosen and release the energy stored in each part of the event. Visualize a slinky toy and how it moves. The tightly coiled spring is looser at each end and coiled tightly in the middle. As the toy moves from one level to another, the spring gradually loosens along its length. This is similar to the way energy is stored in your nervous system after the accident. By "stretching" your accident experience gradually from each end, we drain excess activation, working toward the highest level of energy in the center.

Just Before Your Accident

What was happening in your life just before the accident can have an important bearing on your reaction to it. Events, environment, or states of mind occurring prior to an overwhelming experience such as an auto accident may become fused with the trauma. In other words, if you were feeling relaxed and jubilant before the accident, later you may fear that relaxed and joyous state because you fear that something dangerous will follow it.

Rachel

Rachel was on her way to meet her daughter at a bridal shop to choose a wedding gowns when she had an auto accident. She started her journey happy and excited. After the accident, every time she started to feel happy about something, she panicked.

Through our sessions together, Rachel realized how her feelings of excitement and pleasure just before the accident had become linked in her nervous system with a sense of danger and pain. Once she understood why her feelings of joy and fear had become so overly connected, it only took a short time to help her use resources so that she could feel joy and pleasure once again without fear.

At first, Rachel felt the joy of anticipating her daughter's wedding day, and then panic. In treatment, we helped her see past the accident to remember the wedding and her daughter's happiness today. We worked through the details of the accident to help her discharge the panic. She began to connect the fear appropriately to the oncoming car, not to her sense of joy and expansion.

Take a few minutes to think about the day of your accident: What was your mood? Were you happy? Were you going someplace pleasant? Let's think about that for a minute. How does it make you feel?

- What was your expected outcome of the trip? Your destination or anticipated activities?

- What mood were you in?

- Who were you going to see?

- Who was driving?

- Were there passengers? What was your relationship to them? (Were they family, friends, children, pets?)

- Were there special occasions happening around the time of the accident? (Weddings, births, birthdays, vacations, graduations, family visits?)

- What life stresses were occurring around the time of the accident? (Loss of job or loved one, divorce, bad news, financial problems, moves, trouble with kids?)

- What environmental factors influenced the situation? (Weather conditions, icy roads, visibility problems from sun, fog, rain, shrubbery, trees, kids acting up as a distraction in the car?)

- What resources were in place? (Driving skills, responses, personal support systems, successes, promotions, friendships, personality traits?)

- When was the first instant you were aware something was about to go wrong? Did you have any time to prepare for the threat, or were you blind-sided?

You may need to stop here and do some resiliency exercises.

Evaluating Your Accident

We find the following forms very useful in helping our clients remember the necessary details and examine their feelings about the accident. If you are working with any professionals, you may want to photocopy these forms and take them with you on your next visit. If you are working alone, filling them out may provide some insights into your reactions.

> Remember: Stop if any of the questions make you uncomfortable. You can leave the questions unanswered or continue and do your resourcing exercises.

Client Interview Form

You may wish to fill out the client interview form I use with new clients. Though some of the information here is presented elsewhere, seeing it in this format may help give you a concise overview of your accident.

PRE-ACCIDENT INFORMATION:

Were you driving or were you a passenger, cyclist, or pedestrian?

_____

Where were you going?

_____

How fast?

_____

Were there any other people or pets in the car with you?

_____

How many?

_____

What are/were their names and relationship to you?

_____

_____

_____

Who was driving the car you were in?

_____

The other car?

_____

When did you first perceive that something was wrong?

_____

_____

_____

What emotional state were you in at the time?

_____

What other significant life stressors, if any, were happening at the time of the accident (financial, divorce, family problems, etc.)?

_____

_____

What significant resources, events, or personal support systems are available to you currently?

_____

ACCIDENT INFORMATION:

Please draw a picture of the circumstances in this space. Please mark your car with an X and the other car(s) with #s. Include positions, colors and make of automobiles as well as noting direction, point of impact, damages and speeds of both autos if known.

Please briefly describe what happened, including weather conditions and any special circumstances.

_____

_____

_____

_____

_____

_____

_____

Where did the accident occur?

_____

_____

Time of day?

_____

What do you recall happening to you personally throughout the accident?

_____

_____

_____

_____

_____

_____

_____

_____

Were you wearing a seatbelt? _____ If so, did it feel

Restrictive? _____ Protective?_____ Both? _____

Did an airbag release?

_____

If so, how did that affect you?

_____

_____

Were you injured or did you feel trapped by the seatbelt or airbag?

_____

_____

Were you unconscious at any time?

_____

Any idea how long?

_____

Were you disoriented?

_____

Did you see the other car approaching before impact?

_____

How much time did you have?

_____

During the event, did you have time to respond to the threat or to begin to avoid it?

_____

What do you remember attempting to do?

_____

_____

_____

Do you recall any of your thoughts, emotions, or sensations in your body during the event?

_____

_____

_____

How long did you wait for help to arrive?

_____

How did other drivers or passengers respond?

_____

_____

How did people present at the scene respond?

_____

_____

_____

POST-ACCIDENT INFORMATION:

What was the first thing that happened after the event?

_____

_____

Was it helpful or not?

_____

Did you feel supported?

_____

_____

Threatened?

_____

Other?

_____

Did you experience the police, ambulance, and hospital staff, if involved, to be helpful?

_____

Competent?

_____

Informative?

_____

Any concerns?

_____

_____

When did you begin to feel safer again?

_____

_____

What helps you feel safe now?

_____

_____

Do you feel safe driving since the accident?

_____

What disturbs you the most while driving now?

_____

_____

_____

If there had been enough time, was there anything you were aware of that could have helped to avoid the accident (i.e. honking horns, better visibility, slower speeds, advance warning, etc.)?

_____

_____

_____

_____

Where did you go afterward?

_____

_____

Were you able to rest?

_____

_____

What care have you received?

_____

_____

Are you satisfied with your treatment care?

_____

_____

Who are your current caregivers?

_____

_____

Have you been prescribed medications?

_____

_____

If so, list them with dosages.

_____

_____

_____

Record who is monitoring your medications?

_____

_____

_____

As far as you know, will there be any legal ramifications? _____
If so, describe the situation

_____

_____

_____

_____

What is the outcome you would most like to experience from your
treatment?

_____

_____

_____

Do you have any concerns about treatment?

_____

_____

_____

_____

Draw on the body pictures below to locate and mark any of your current injuries since the auto accident, including ongoing or intermittent pain, tension, or numbing patterns. Indicate previous injuries that you have had or ones that may have been exacerbated since the accident.

Body Map

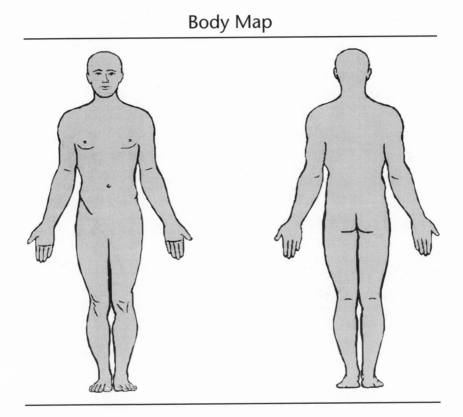

PREVIOUS AUTO ACCIDENT AND MEDICAL HISTORY:

Describe any pre-existing conditions you had prior to this accident.

_____

_____

_____

Have you had any accidents with similar circumstances before?

_____

_____

Have you had other auto accidents?_____ List dates and brief descriptions:

_____

_____

_____

ADDITIONAL INFORMATION FOR SYMPTOM EVALUATION:

Did you experience, witness, or encounter an event in which there was *perceived or actual* threat to the life of yourself or others?

_____

_____

Threat of physical injury to yourself or others?

_____

_____

Were there any injuries or fatalities? Describe:

_____

_____

Did you experience intense fear, helplessness, or horror?

_____

_____

Do you experience recurrent and intrusive distressing recollections of the event, including images, thoughts, or perceptions?

_____

_____

_____

Do you experience recurrent distressing dreams of the event?

_____

_____

Do you experience acting or feeling as if the traumatic event were recurring?

_____

_____

Do you experience psychological distress upon exposure to triggers that remind you of the accident?

_____

_____

Do you experience physiological reactivity or activation when triggered by events or circumstances that remind you of the accident?

_____

_____

Do you experience hyperarousal at:

Intersections? _____ Stoplights? _____

Cars approaching you from certain directions? Which directions?

_____

_____

Heavy traffic?

_____

Specific weather conditions? Explain.

_____

_____

Merge lanes?

_____

Do you experience:

Anger at other drivers?

_____

Avoidance of location of accident?

_____

Reactions to similar make, model, or color of the auto that hit you?

_____

_____

Other driving difficulties?

_____

_____

Do you try to avoid memories, or conversations associated with the accident?

_____

_____

Do you try to avoid activities, such as driving, or places such as the location of the accident?

_____

_____

Do you have difficulty remembering aspects of the accident?

_____

_____

Do you feel an incessant need to tell your story?

_____

_____

Do you participate in important activities less often than before the accident?

_____

Do you feel isolated or disconnected from others?

_____

_____

Do you notice a lack of emotional responsiveness? (i.e. unable to have loving feelings, unable to feel pleasure, unable to cry, etc.)

_____

_____

Do you feel a sense of a foreboding about the future?

_____

Are you afraid the accident will happen again?

_____

Do you experience irritability or exaggerated frustration or uncontrollable rage?

_____

Do you feel easily distracted or preoccupied?

_____

Do you experience hypervigilant or overcautious?

_____

Do you experience an exaggerated startle response or feel jumpy?

_____

Has the accident disrupted your functioning at work or socially?

_____

_____

The duration of these symptoms has been:

_____ Less than 3 months (acute) _____ More than 3 months (chronic)

_____ Symptoms begin at least 6 months after the accident (delayed reaction)

The Importance of Context

Your reaction to the accident stems from more than just the accident events, or what actually happened during the accident. You also need to evaluate what else was going on in your life.

If everything else was perfect, the accident caused little or no injury, the paramedics were helpful, and the insurance company paid promptly, then your accident may be resolved quite easily. More likely you were dealing with other life stresses—family problems, financial problems, or job worries. Three of David Rippe's family members died in the months preceding his accident. You need to acknowledge these other stresses and identify the supports available to you. The accident itself may be less upsetting than the context in which it happened. Perhaps your accident occurred in a rural area and it was hours before help arrived. The whole picture of what is happening in your life affects your reactions.

If you were in the car with children or pets at the time of the accident, often you need to take time to deal with your feelings and reactions about them as part of your healing process before you can focus fully on your own recovery.

Exercise: What If?

This exercise helps you substitute "what if" scenarios for the events of your accident.

What would have happened if you had gotten there as scheduled? Imagine yourself arriving safely at your original destination. Who would you like to be there with you? What would your reactions have been? When was the first time you felt safe afterward?

Now move to the very first "Oh, no!" moment—the first instant when you realized the accident was about to happen and notice your physical reaction. What if you had had time to turn out of the way?

By focusing on the resources that you have and imagining a positive outcome, you establish "solid ground" or oasis at the beginning and end of the accident. As you think about the accident, return to these positive resources over and over until you gain a feeling of safety and control. Shifting back and forth from accident scenes to resources interrupts the physiological pattern that got established during the accident. It helps break the pattern and discharge the survival energy that has mobilized.

> Remember: You are present and alive now. If you feel your body becoming tense or your breathing gets fast, loop back into your resources. Think of someone who is comforting and helpful to you. Imagine them there with you. Remember how feeling safe feels in your body.

Linking—Why You May Be Afraid of White Cars

Remember how we talked earlier in this chapter about how emotions or events you experienced at the time of the accident can become fused with the accident itself? These associations are called "linking."

Linking develops because of the way the reptilian brain functions. Because the reptilian brain responds very quickly to threat, without taking time to differentiate exactly which of the many things you are experiencing is the actual threat, it simply takes a mental snapshot of everything happening. This includes the weather conditions, the color of the car that hit you, the yellow or red light, or barking dogs nearby. After the accident, anything included in that snapshot may become a danger signal to you, retriggering your fear and anxiety. This explains why you may feel terrified whenever you see a white car, if a white car hit you, or, why you start to panic when someone is pulling up behind you if you were previously rear-ended. One of the most common forms of linking is the location of the accident. Many people get very eerie feelings when they pass the spot where their accident took place. Others will go to great lengths never to drive by the accident site again.

These triggers can take you right back into the trauma of the accident, much as a Vietnam veteran may be mentally transported back to his war experiences by the sounds of a helicopter flying overhead or a car backfiring. This is an unconscious reaction that cannot be overcome by your rational brain, no matter how often you tell your-self you are in no danger from that white car pulling up behind you.

Often, until you have worked through the various phases of the accident, you don't realize your brain has linked so many outside events to your accident. Once you can understand and unlink them, many of the unusual fears that may have plagued you since your accident will vanish.

Cynthia

Cynthia rode her bicycle to work every day. Biking was more than trans-portation to her; much of her recreational activity focused on it. One day, while rushing to work, peddling along in the bike lane with her head down, she crashed face-first into a garbage truck parked in the bike lane. She suffered serious facial wounds and needed plastic surgery.

Cynthia's first reaction was to give up cycling completely. She never wanted to bike again. As she worked through her fears, she was able to begin to ride again, but for many months was unable to take a direct route to work, circling many blocks out of her way to avoid the accident site. She also became extremely safety-conscious. Whenever she saw others riding without helmets, she became angry and chided them for their care-lessness.

After a number of sessions, Cynthia regained her enjoyment of biking, but it took many more sessions before she overcame the terror she felt every time she saw a garbage truck.

Drawing Your Accident Helps

Use the following diagram to help you draw your accident and any previous accidents you might have had. Drawing the accident may help you remember some details you had forgotten, and when we begin to work on boundary rupture and whiplash it gives you a visual record of which side the impact came from. This will help you work through your personal fears or injuries. You need to know what happened to your body and where it happened.

Accident Chart and Timeline

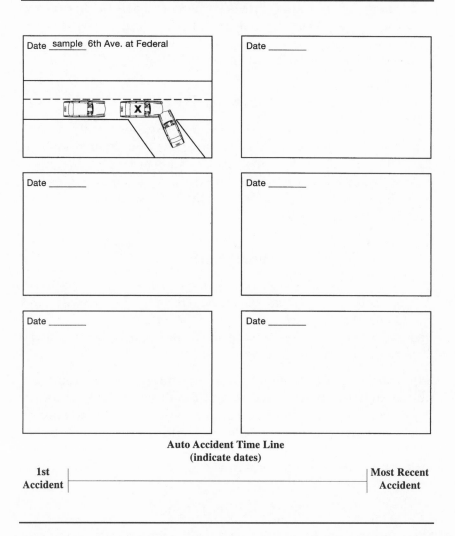

Date <u>sample</u> 6th Ave. at Federal

Date _____

Date _____

Date _____

Date _____

Date _____

Auto Accident Time Line
(indicate dates)

| 1st Accident | | Most Recent Accident |

Whenever you begin to feel stressed during this process, stop and do your resourcing exercises.

Now recall the specific circumstances of each accident.

Did someone run a stoplight? Was there ice or snow that caused your car to slide? Were you rear-ended at a stop sign? Write down and draw what happened. Remember to refer to resources or change your focus if this exercise is anxiety producing.

Simultaneous Threats

You might have had to deal with two simultaneous threats. It's natural for your eyes to lock onto one threat at a time. Your vision narrows when you locate an initial threat, making a second threat easy to miss. For instance, you might have had two cars approaching you from different directions, or you might have been blinded by the sun while merging into traffic.

Marybeth

Marybeth was carefully driving through a complicated construction zone. Ahead, she saw a gravel truck pulling onto the road. She focused on this danger and was completely stunned when she crashed into another, closer truck pulling into her path. "How could I be so stupid as to miss seeing a truck? It was enormous!" she kept repeating.

Often survivors of accidents involving simultaneous threats feel humiliation and shame because they didn't see the second threat. They need to understand that this is a natural result of the body's reaction to danger. They were focused entirely on the first threat they saw. Their field of vision narrowed. It was physically impossible for them to see the second threat.

How Did You React?

Did you honk your horn? Simply learning where your horn is and training yourself to use it gives you greater driving safety. Did you signal, or slow down? Did you try to turn out of the way? Did you slam on the brakes?

Memory Gaps

Do you have memory gaps, or were you unconscious after the accident? Memory gaps are common after accidents. You often will regain these memories as the energy in your body is released. As I explained in Chapter 5 on logjamming, your body is protecting you from the overload of too much stimulus. Your memory has become fragmented. As excess energy is released, the fragmentation is reduced. The gaps fill in as you reconnect to body awareness. Trauma memory becomes internalized in the body. As you progress in your work on the sensation level, you are likely to regain most of your memory.

When you find yourself unable to remember a portion of the accident, it indicates the activation level in your body was too high. Trauma survivors often experience having intact memory to a certain point, then there is no recall available. Soon memory picks up again. We refer to these as "memory markers" on each side of the gap.

Jeremy

After a serious collision, Jeremy suffered a memory loss. His last memory marker before the accident was a memory of briefly glancing up at planes overhead in an air show. The next thing he remembered was waking up in the hospital after surgery for a head injury. As we reviewed his shift in attention away from driving to the synchronized jets and gave him time, he recalled seeing a red Honda in his peripheral vision, swerving into his lane from the left. I had him imagine staring at the jets and feeling the thrill he felt watching them. Then I had him switch focus to see only the red Honda.

I suggested he freeze-frame, or mentally stop the Honda as far away from him as he needed to feel that looking at it was manageable. He felt a wave of relief move through him as he had time to locate the threat and "see what had hit him" for the first time. Then his body had time to recognize survival plans he didn't have time to access or act on originally. With more time he might have swerved out of the way or honked his horn. We expanded time to allow him to feel his hands on the wheel and organize his turning to get out of the way successfully. We had him listen to the loud sound of his horn and feel the pressure of his hand on it. He felt stronger. Even though he hadn't had time to take these actions when his accident happened, it felt empowering to him to rehearse and play them out now in the session.

It was a relief to Jeremy to remember and be aware of more of the story. He began to remember that he had argued with his son that morning, and that he had been angry and more distracted than usual while he was driving. Having survived the accident and the surgery, he and his son had reconciled. His body relaxed further when he touched into the harmony he now experienced with his child.

Next Jeremy began to feel the force of the collision move through the car and his body. He imagined a childhood experience in bumper cars at an amusement park that had the effect of softening the blow. He had been in control of the bumper car, and collisions were intentional and tolerable. He felt the contrast of being caught off guard and out of control with being in charge and having fun. Again his body let down. He heard the sound of honking his horn again, which felt like he was saying "no," or giving warning to the other driver.

Then Jeremy remembered the siren of the ambulance that had taken him to the hospital. Again, he felt initially activated by the memory but then relief at recalling what had happened. He began to recall the feeling of being strapped down on the ambulance gurney and the soothing and reassuring voice of the paramedic talking to him. He felt his arms wanting to break through the straps that were holding him down. He felt strong and powerful.

During surgery, Jeremy had anesthesia, which gave him a double layer of forced amnesia. While he is not likely to regain memories of the surgery itself, many clients do recall being in the operating room and recovery room as their memory returns.

After surgery, Jeremy woke up to the supportive faces of his wife and son. In our session, he felt the hangover drowsiness of the anesthesia and could smell hospital smells. He began to connect more and more of the events before, during, and after the accident and hospitalization.

It's not necessary to recall every detail of your accident. You just need to remember enough to reestablish a sense of continuity so that you realize you actually went through the experience and that it is now over. That allows you to move on.

The steps you need to take during your exercises, as Jeremy did in his sessions, are:

- Noticing how you first experienced the threat

- Allowing completion of defensive orienting—review your alternative survival strategies, i.e. swerving, honking your horn, breaking the straps on the gurney

- Adding corrective experience—imagining a similar, but pleasant experience (i.e. bumper cars)

- Reviewing your resources—(for Jeremy, the resolution with his son, giving himself time, remembering reassuring paramedics)

- Filling in memory gaps.

How much warning time did you have before the accident? Did you see it coming? Was there time to respond? What did you do? The less time you had to respond, the more activating the experience will be for you.

Olivia

When the car Olivia was riding in collided with another, she was thrown from the back seat across the front and into the windshield. Describing her accident, she said, "When I hit the windshield, I felt as if time and space collapsed."

After the accident, Olivia constantly felt as if she was rushing urgently from one place to another. She never had enough time in her day. At the same time, she was unable to arrive anywhere on time. Her constant tardiness jeopardized her job.

"I try so hard to be on time," she said. "I'll look at the clock and it's five minutes to 8:00. The next time I look, it's 9:15, and I have no idea where the time has gone."

It is quite common for accident survivors to have problems similar to Olivia's. Your sense of time is compromised. This can endanger jobs and relationships when those around you can't understand that there is a physiological reason for your inability to manage time.

Exercise: Adding Time

This is another exercise to give you the sense of having enough time.

Visualize that "Oh, no" moment again. Now imagine time slowing down. Mentally take the other car and place it a safe distance away. Keep it there. This is what we've discussed as freeze-framing, or stopping the image. Where is that for you? A block away? Miles away? Imagine seeing that car and having your "Oh, no" moment from this new distance. You can see the threat while having the resources of time and space. What happens in your body? Does your breathing slow? Mentally look around you at the accident site. Do you see things you didn't notice before? Is there someplace that would have been safe to steer your car if you had had time to make a decision? Imagine your car going there now, before the other car reaches you.

Accidents give us so little response time that we may not realize how appropriate our reactions were. Slowing down the process in your mind gives you time to look at your reaction and to understand it. It gives you space to let your body reorganize and complete survival plans that you didn't have time for at the moment of the accident.

You may feel trapped in the moment of the accident, unable to move forward with your life. One of the signs that the trauma is resolving is the sense that the accident is moving back into the past, into its proper position in time. You feel that it is over and you can be present in your life now and have faith in the future.

If you are still unable to visualize removing the other car as a threat or slowing the accident down, return to the earlier resourcing exercises. Use the beginning exercise of feeling your body in the chair. Keep reminding yourself that you survived, that what you did worked and no matter how you reacted, you succeeded.

- Were you wearing a seatbelt? Did it help you feel protected, or did you feel trapped? Did your airbag deploy? Chapter 13 will take you through exercises to overcome any trauma you may have from seatbelts or airbags.

- What specific difficulties did you experience? These might include going through the windshield, having your brakes fail, hitting the steering wheel, having the other driver yell at you, or worries about children or pets in the car.

- What specific advantages or resources did you experience? Did a guardrail prevent your car from going into the river? Did you hit a snow bank that protected you?

After the Accident

Next, we will work with events after the accident. Remember that working through the accident chronologically activates your nervous system and can cause additional stress. Don't be tempted to charge forward and get through the whole thing all at once.

Events after the accident might have either contributed to the intensity of your experience or reduced it. As you work through this portion of the accident, stop frequently to loop back to your resources, and to do exercises envisioning a different outcome to the experience.

- What happened immediately after the accident? Was there someone there to help? Were other people at the scene calm and helpful? Were the paramedics kind and reassuring? One client was screaming in panic when the paramedics slapped an oxygen mask over her face to quiet her, increasing her trauma. Others have had very positive experiences, with paramedics who held their hands and talked softly, reassuring them that things would be okay.

Even in relatively minor accidents, other people's reactions surrounding the event may be so devastating that your response is more linked to lack of environmental support than to the accident itself.

Rosemary

Rosemary skidded on ice. Her car struck a light pole. She was frightened, but not hurt. When she got home, her father reacted to the accident by becoming extremely agitated and rageful, and blaming of her. He said she should have been able to avoid the accident, should have been more cautious, should have taken a different route. Rosemary began to have anxiety attacks when she was driving. For her, the most traumatic piece was not the accident, but her father's reaction.

As she and I explored her father's strange reactions, we learned that when he was young, he and his younger brother were in the car when their parents had an accident. His younger brother was killed. Rosemary's accident triggered a powerful traumatic memory for him.

Such extreme and inappropriate reactions are often symptomatic of unresolved trauma.

When I had my accident, not only was the other driver physically unharmed, but also an oral surgeon, meaning that he was able to help with my injuries immediately and calmly.

You may have experienced conflict with the other driver, felt isolated and alone, or blamed yourself or others. Having the presence of someone supportive can be invaluable at a time like this.

Exercise: Post-Accident Actions

Imagining how you wish things had happened can be soothing.

Imagine yourself immediately after the accident. Who was there? What did they do that you found helpful. If no one was available, who would you have wanted to be with you if possible? Imagine what they would have done to help. How does this help you feel safe? Take your time with this feeling until you can feel it having a positive effect on your body. When you feel your resources having a positive effect on your body, give yourself plenty of time to enjoy that relaxation response and to notice the details of how and where your body is relaxing.

How was your experience with the ambulance and hospital emergency service? Were they supportive and informed? Did they make you feel safe? If support after the accident was effective, then we want you to feel the sense of relief and being well cared for.

If support was lacking in an area, we'd like you to switch focus to what you would have preferred. What did you need from the medical team? If it was comforting words, write down what they would be. Repeat them aloud to yourself now. How do you feel hearing the right kind of support?

Even though the support you actually did receive may have felt inade-quate, something inside you—your own blueprint for health—knows what would have been right. You can trust your body's intelligence about what it needed.

When did you first begin to feel safe again? When help arrived? When you saw a familiar face? When you arrived at the hospital or at home? When someone you love held you? Perhaps a friend brought you a blanket and a cup of tea.

Take a moment to experience this feeling of safety again. How does it feel in your body? Do you feel warm? Comforted? Return to this feeling whenever you need to feel safe.

Accident Aftermaths

Inevitably, you have suffered losses as a result of your accident. David Rippe suffered chronic migraines for three years. Susan nearly had to drop out of graduate school because she was unable to work. One client, a dentist, lost the hand-eye coordination necessary for his career. Another, a massage therapist, suffered a shoulder injury and had to leave her practice.

Discharging excess energy can do a great deal to relieve symptoms, but there may be injuries requiring further surgery or other treatment. Work to establish a network of supportive professionals and friends to give you a support system during this time.

Changes or losses in your job, relationships, overall health, and financial status may be permanent. You will experience grief over these losses. It is important to allow yourself to grieve.

We do not mean to minimize these changes in your life in any way. We encourage creative new possibilities that are open to you, rather than dwelling on the negative. For instance, the massage therapist used her accident settlement to return to school and now is a successful psychotherapist. In the middle of your present crisis, it is difficult to see how something positive can come from your accident, but as you work through this book, you will see how many others have experienced important positive life changes.

It is interesting to note that the Chinese use the same symbol for both crisis and opportunity.

Key Points

- Your accident should not be worked on or retold chronologically, as that can be retraumatizing

- Start working on your accident by remembering the first time you felt safe *after* the accident

- What was happening in your life before the accident is important

- Because accidents usually happen very quickly, inserting time to stretch out the experience of your accident is crucial

- The overall context of your life, previous traumas, level of stress, and childhood history comes into play in the aftermath of your accident

- Real losses as a result of your accident need to be grieved

10

◇

Boundary Rupture and Repair

> Note: Be sure any professional you may be working with reads and understands this chapter. It can be very counterproductive and unnecessarily traumatic for your physical therapist to work in your wounded boundary area until it has been repaired. As you read through this chapter you will understand why.

Personal Boundaries

The concept of personal boundaries may be new to you, but the feeling of having your space invaded isn't. Have you ever talked to someone who stood so close that you wanted to take a step back? Subconsciously, you were aware that they were in your personal space. Each of us has a sense of our own space, a space surrounded by energetic boundaries. When someone invades these boundaries, we feel uncomfortable.

Boundaries help us contain our internal experience so that we are not flooded with excessive emotion. Boundaries also buffer us from too much stimulus or a sense of invasion from the outside. Just like we need our physical skin to define inside and outside, we use energetic boundaries to define our personal space. We are upset when we cut our skin; we are upset when we feel our boundaries are ruptured or compromised.

When we have intact boundaries we can filter stimulus or shift attention away from something annoying, such as the sound of a loudly ticking clock. We also instinctively know to move away from a person or a situation that feels toxic or invasive to us. Boundaries help us feel a sense of personal safety in the world. Normally people experience a sense of 360 degrees of containment much like being inside a protective sphere or safe energetic envelope.

Boundaries are flexible depending on the situation. If a friend or loved one is approaching us we usually feel that they can come in close to us to the point of physical contact, such as a handshake or a hug. If someone is a stranger and feels dangerous to us we obviously need much more distance and our boundaries may feel quite dense and rigid until we have established the distance we need. When we have developed boundary sensitivity we can also tell how much distance we need in any given situation. We can sense when someone has moved too close and know to shift our position. One sign that our boundaries are intact and functioning occurs when we can discern the need for space and distance in varying circumstances.

In my classes, I demonstrate how difficult it is to feel any sense of containment when boundaries are ruptured. I hold a sieve above a bowl and pour water through it. The sieve represents damaged non-functional boundaries and the bowl intact ones. The water represents experience or stimulus. There is not much use in trying to work with the trauma until you can hold and integrate the healing. This demonstration dramatically shows the importance of boundary repair in the treatment process.

In our classes on auto accident recovery we do an exercise that helps people experience their sense of boundaries, both where they feel in place and where there is a rupture. Once we had a high-ranking officer in the armed forces in our class. He was a very muscular, brush-cut former paratrooper who was skeptical about this concept of boundaries. I invited him to be a participant in an exercise.

I simply had him imagine himself within a protective sphere. I had him focus specifically on which direction felt the safest—for him, in front. His second most secure section was behind him. As he imagined the sector on his left side he felt some anxiety, but when he began exploring the sector to his right he immediately had an image of being struck by a truck from the right in an auto accident five years earlier.

As we explored that sector further, even more images came up for him about being wounded on that side in battle. To watch this very tough soldier allow his vulnerability and emotion to surface in the group was very moving for all of us. The exercise further demonstrated that boundaries have nothing to do with strength of character, but reflect an energetic reality.

After my accident, I "lost left." I couldn't look left without consciously moving my head in that direction. I couldn't bear to be approached from the left. Even today, I recognize that I am more sensitive to people standing close to me on that side than I am to people in other parts of my personal space.

In an auto accident, our boundaries can be ruptured, leaving us feeling undefended. If the boundary rupture is severe, we may lose our feeling of containment. Boundary rupture symptoms include:

- A raw feeling of walking around without your skin

- Hypersensitivity to sound, light, or touch

- A lack of defenses or ability to filter stimulus

- Feeling like you are flooding out into your surroundings, or that they are flooding in on you

- A tendency to re-injure yourself in a particular area, or being accident-prone.

Since we don't usually think of ourselves in terms of being contained by boundaries, the feeling of boundary rupture can be very puzzling. Until you can repair your ruptured boundaries, you will not feel a full sense of safety and completeness. You can be retraumatized by people approaching you from areas of boundary rupture, and not understand your fear.

Exercise: Checking for Boundary Rupture

The goal of this exercise is to test for any areas of boundary rupture.

Try this exercise with a friend. Sit in a chair. Have the friend approach you from directly in front. How does that feel? Now have her approach from directly behind. Does that disturb you at all? Repeat the exercise with your friend approaching from each side. If you have had a boundary rupture in any area, you will find it uncomfortable or even frightening to be approached from that direction.

Have your friend approach from the ruptured area more slowly. Does this feel less threatening? Where do you want her to stop? At first you may want her to take small steps and stop many feet away.

When she gets as close as is comfortable, have her stop. Notice what it feels like to define your boundary and have it respected. Does this resource make you feel more at ease? How would it feel in your body to know someone was there to protect you? Do you notice a relaxation response? Keep repeating the exercise and the shift to a resource until you do not feel threatened by someone in that area of your personal space.

It is very important to let any healthcare or bodyworkers know about your boundary rupture so that they can approach you from a different direction or sit in a position that doesn't threaten you. After doing boundary repair work, one of our clients reported how she came to the realization that every time her chiropractor worked on her neck, she became activated and anxious. Even though the chiropractor had excellent technique, it wasn't until our client healed her boundary rupture that her work with the chiropractor became most productive.

Your boundaries might have been ruptured in more than one spot. Pull out the sketch you did of your accident. Did the other car strike you from the left? If so, it's likely that your boundary is ruptured on the left. But because your body was forced to the right and you might have struck something or had whiplash, your right boundary may be ruptured as well. A rear-end collision that forces you into the steering wheel will rupture front and back boundaries.

Study this sample this pie chart and use it as a model to map where your boundaries are ruptured and where they are intact. Don't forget that your boundaries are actually three-dimensional. You may also feel danger from above or below.

Points of Rupture

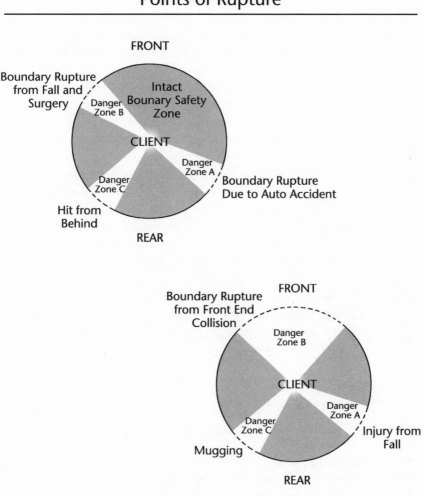

Exercise: Evaluating Boundary Rupture

The goal of this exercise is to help you further evaluate your boundary rupture. It was originally designed by Darrell Sanchez, a Rolfer and trauma recovery specialist in Boulder, Colorado.

Imagine that you are sitting or standing in a sphere. Gradually become aware of all 360 degrees around you. Try to sense the direction where you feel the safest and most protected so we can determine where your boundaries are most intact. This helps you become aware of what boundaries feel like energetically and to discover how you experience safety and protection in your body. Always start from where the boundaries feel most intact and build from strength. You may be astonished how exact you are in detecting the specific line of demarcation between what feels safe spatially and where the lack of safety begins. You may be able to literally draw a line in space once your attention is focused in this area. When you work with a therapist, it is important to make sure that the area they are sitting in does not coincide with your area of boundary rupture. If they do sit in this area, you may have a sense of danger or activation rather than feeling helped by their presence. Or you may prefer them there.

To continue the exercise, examine the next safest direction. Find resources to strengthen that area. How would your body want to add protection? Would it like a shield or the presence of a friendly protective ally? As that direction gets stronger and you feel safe, go on to explore the next area until eventually you feel supported and safe from all directions. As we target certain directions, my clients often remember different traumatic experiences they've encountered and thought were already resolved. This exercise reveals important information that only tapping into the boundary awareness seems to be able to provide.

Rita

Rita, a building inspector, stood up abruptly and injured her head on a beam. For the next several months she repeatedly bumped her head on things above her. She was baffled by her sudden clumsiness.

When she came to me for help, I showed her how her initial injury cre-

ated a boundary rupture, making her unable to orient properly to danger from above. Because her reptilian brain had identified "up" as danger-ous, it blocked that area from her awareness repertoire. She wasn't able to include "up" in her inventory of safe places. After some boundary repair exercises, Rita regained her normal caution about overhead objects. She could sense them and avoid hitting her head.

Repairing the Damage

You'll start working from your safest point to repair boundary rup-ture. You'll draw on all the resources you need, both real and imag-inary, to restore your sense of containment.

Exercise: Finding Safety Zones

This exercise helps you assess your safety zones, and convert your boundary rupture into body sensation.

What direction feels safest? Where does your sense of safety shift? Where does the danger zone start? What does it feel like? (One client described the area of impact as feeling like a huge metal door was slamming on her when she oriented there.)

What kind of resource might your body want there? Someone to defend you? A shield? Something soft and shock absorbing like pillows? Take a moment to let your body feel each of these options. How do they feel? Are you feeling a sense of expansion or trembling that signifies discharge of energy? Think of your intact boundaries as a safety zone that allows the discharge of excess activation as you move back and forth between the safe and danger areas. It is often useful to just touch the edge of where the activation begins, like putting your toe into water and then back out again.

As the trapped energy begins to discharge, your boundaries will fill in the areas of rupture and repair themselves. It is natural for your body to heal boundaries as your resiliency increases. Continue with your resourcing exercises, imagining resources that protect you from the feelings of rupture, until you no longer experience apprehen-sion when someone approaches.

Repaired Boundaries

When your boundaries are intact, you should experience a sense of enhanced safety. You may feel you are protected by an energetic bubble that surrounds and contains you. Body boundaries feel flexible in density and distance from the body, and they discriminate between safety and danger.

Key Points

- We all have personal boundaries

- Boundaries filter both internal and external experiences

- Trauma can create a breach in those boundaries

- That breach makes us vulnerable to more trauma

- Boundaries can be repaired, becoming intact again as the energy mobilized to deal with threat is discharged

11

Impact!

You've practiced your resourcing exercises. You've worked on the events before and after the accident, releasing energy and discharging activation. You know how to avoid becoming overactivated from dealing with accident details, and you're learning how to repair your boundary ruptures. Now it's time to work toward the actual moment of impact.

Remembering Your Accident

Don't be distressed if you can't remember everything about your accident. Some parts, especially the moment of impact, are likely to be fragmented because of how highly activated these memories are. As you release the energy, more and more of your memory will return.

You may feel an inclination to rush into this portion of the work to get through it. Don't be tempted to do so. If you move ahead too quickly you can cause yourself to disconnect or start to flood. You may find that you have a powerful avoidance of the material because it is so strongly charged. Again, moving one step at a time will help you through this difficult portion of your recovery.

> REMEMBER: This material can be highly stressful. Work slowly, and return to your resources often.

Getting Ready

Practice your resourcing exercises again before you start this phase of work. Be sure that you are able to stop and back out if you become activated. You may encounter unexpectedly strong emotions when dealing with this portion of the work. Be sure your resources are fully in place so that you can work bit by bit to slowly release the energy.

Softening the Impact

The first thing we'll do is work to soften the impact in your memory with some exercises.

Exercise: Kinesthetic Softening

The purpose of this exercise is to replace the actual impact in your memory with a softer experience. This provides a competing physiological experience that helps to neutralize the impact.

Think of your accident. Imagine that instead of being metal, your car and the other car were encased in pillows. Now think how that would feel when the two cars came together. How might it have changed what happened to your body?

What if your car and the other car had been carnival bumper cars, hitting one another deliberately. Remember what fun that was when you were a child? What does it feel like in your body when you think of choosing small impacts while being in control and safe?

Continue doing this exercise, substituting other items for your metal car. What if they had been stuffed cars, foam balls, clouds, or feathers? How does that change what happens in your body?

Exercise: Auditory Softening

Many of my clients report that the loud noise of the impact is what they remember and find most distressing. Remember David in Chapter 8, whose only memory of his accident was the sound of glass breaking? This exercise helps substitute another experience for the sound of the accident.

Think of your accident. Recall the sound of impact. Now, imagine that you were wearing earplugs when the accident happened. What happens in your body when the sound is muffled?

Touch into the sound of impact again. Now think of hearing music you particularly love. Hear the music playing throughout the moment of impact. What happens in your body when the sound you hear is beautiful? Notice how your chest feels. What happens in your heart? In your stomach? Your shoulders and arms?

Exercise: Visual Softening

Accidents happen so quickly that your nervous system doesn't have time to complete the threat response. Also, other images become linked with your memory of the accident through your reptilian brain's snapshot reaction to a trauma scene. This exercise helps slow down the events and defuse the intrusive images.

Remember the exercise you practiced in the resource chapter to slow the accident down? Let's work through it again. Imagine that the other car is a safe distance away. Now imagine that the other car is moving toward you very slowly. You can stop it and give yourself time to look at it whenever you need to. Freeze-frame the image of the car to see how your body responds with the threat at bay and with time to react. Notice the intelligence of your body's survival plans. Let yourself give into them.

How does it feel in your body if you turn your car out of the way? How does it feel if you jump out of your car and run to a safe spot? Pay attention to what's happening in your body. What if you could reach out and push the other car away before it hits yours? How does this feel physically?

REMEMBER: We can't change history, but we can allow the body to relax. The danger is over. Completing these imaginary responses helps you let go of unnecessary tension.

Lil

Lil came to us nearly a year after her accident because she was having anxiety about driving and had a great deal of anger at the driver who cut her off and caused her accident. She didn't feel the need to remember the impact. She could recall seeing the black van cut in front of her, then nothing. The next thing she remembered was her car being pointed in a different direction.

Initially she felt extremely disoriented and angry with the other driver, who had been reckless. Lil had injured her hand and wrist, and needed surgery. The hand still caused extreme pain. Fortunately she'd had excellent medical care at the scene of the accident and afterward.

Lil had completed parts of her accident experience by inserting time for her to react and feel more in control. For example, she fantasized pushing the offending car out of the way, or driving a large army tank so strong that the other car just bounced off without harming her. Both images represent completing a thwarted fight response and helped resolve her anger. Going through these images gave her nervous system a chance to discharge.

Then I had her visualize the black van again. When we inserted the resource of time, Lil felt her body want to speed up and continue on her way or to swerve of the highway to safety on the shoulder. These reflected versions represent completing her thwarted flight responses. After each completion she relaxed more and breathed more easily.

Still, Lil had little or no memory of the impact. Her hand and wrist regained function after the surgery, but they still felt separate from her body—an example of a body part being dissociated. Since dissociation indicates high activation we knew we had more work to do.

Lil wanted to "steer clear" of re-experiencing the impact, so we did it very slowly with many breaks where we accessed resources. She felt she couldn't see, then realized once she knew collision was imminent she had closed her eyes. She could feel she had her glasses on but could feel her eyelids squeezed shut.

She sensed where her hands were on the steering wheel at seven and three o'clock. I had her imagine gripping the wheel tighter to help her feel the wheel even more. Then she released it and more activation was discharged.

Lil said suddenly, "My hands are back. They ache, but they're back. Oh, my God, I know how the injury happened now."

She could remember her hand and wrist twisting inside the steering wheel and hitting the steering column at impact. She felt the force of being shoved off the highway by the black van. As sensory motor mem-

ory came back she felt high activation followed by relief as confusion cleared.

Lil suddenly realized what a close call it had been and felt a surge of anxiety. She also felt tremendous fear about being hit a second time in highway traffic or from behind after stopping, because her car stopped before the black van did. I had her take time to take it in that she had not been hit a second time. Once her car had stopped she'd been safe. Together we returned to the original impact and this time touching into it felt smoother and more pieces came together. She felt more and more connected and integrated. The pieces fit and the memory felt right to her.

She began to see more of the whole picture. She could see her dashboard, the steering wheel, the windshield, the guardrail, and the other car. I had her look at each piece individually to help her orient. She looked up toward the mountains in the distance and felt she could touch them to ground herself. She said she could remember how it had all happened so fast, but now that she had survived, she had time to sort it all out. As each piece filled in, Lil felt relief. She felt joyful and exhilarated in the fact that she had survived. She felt she could explore her surroundings.

She said she felt that she was choosing this new direction herself (the one she had been forced into by the collision.) She wanted to be in this place. She scanned her body inside and her surroundings outside and everything felt just fine.

Overcoming Freeze

The most common response at the moment of impact is to freeze. After all, there isn't much option! You're strapped in, with no time to unhook your seatbelt and run, much less fight back.

When you begin to work on your feeling of being frozen, you may have a fairly strong reaction. It's typical when freeze response begins to release that you will move into the fight-or-flight response. You may want to run or feel like hitting someone. You may feel violently angry toward the other driver. This violent or intense impulse is natural because of the amount of energy trapped in your nervous system. Allow yourself to feel the impulse and see the image. Notice what happens in your body when you do. Having the thought does not mean that you have become a violent person. We encourage you to allow the anger energy to move through in a way that is safe for you and others rather than to act out.

Your cognitive brain will try to override your reptilian brain. You may feel guilty about expressing anger. (Women tend to have more guilt feelings about anger than men do.) Anger is a natural part of the incomplete fight-or-flight response; part of the life-saving system built into your reptilian brain.

Cynthia

Cynthia, the person we talked about earlier who rode her bicycle into a garbage truck, had a lot of suppressed anger, especially triggered when she saw these trucks. I had her visualize walking up to the truck, starting from as far away as she wanted. She chose to start from several blocks back. I asked her to visualize to the truck and notice where it was parked— something she didn't have time to do during the accident. She began to feel a sense of threat.

I then asked Cynthia how her body wanted to respond to the threat. She said she would like to smash the truck, so she visualized herself doing that. Next she wanted to hit the driver. She imagined doing so, paying close attention to her body sensations and reported that it felt good. She felt less helpless and more powerful. In my experience, imagining options gives the body much relief. I certainly don't advocate actually acting out the violence!

Larry

My husband, Larry, was almost rear-ended by a sports utility vehicle (SUV). As he continued on his errand, he suddenly realized that SUVs surrounded him. Suddenly they seemed to be everywhere, and he realized he was angry with all of them! Even in this example of a near miss, you can see how experiencing threat can activate a fight response and how the reptilian brain can globalize danger.

Exercise: Fight Response

This exercise helps you deal with your normal impulse to fight. In the past, therapists often had their patients actually hit one another with foam bats or beat a pillow to discharge anger. We've learned that there is more energy discharged in the process of organizing to act, which you do when you envision scenarios, than in the actual movements.

Imagine that you are about to hit the other driver. Do an internal scan of your body. As you imagine yourself preparing to strike out, feel how your body organizes itself to do so. Notice what happens in your muscles when you get ready for action. Feel yourself completing the action in slow motion. What happens in your body? Many clients report that sensing the completion of the fight response facilitates a deep relief.

Exercise: Flight Response

Picture yourself running away from the accident. What happens in your body? What are your legs feeling? How does it feel to escape from the accident? Where do you want to run to? What happens when you find a safe place?

After trauma, we lose our awareness of how it feels to prepare to act. These exercises will help you regain the sensation of preparatory motion. Awareness of these motions facilitates a much deeper release than acting out would.

Moving Through Impact

Remember that you already have survived the accident. No matter what happens as you are working back through the events, you already have accomplished the most difficult part. Yes, you may still have symptoms, but what you did at the time of the accident worked. You are alive.

Working through the life-threatening moment of impact may take several attempts. The more threatening your experience, the more traumatic it was. Keep reminding yourself that though you may have nearly died, you did not. You survived.

Exercise: Discharging the Activation of Impact

The only way to release activation from the impact and complete your recovery is to deal with the event. But just like we did with events at the beginning of the accident and at the end, we are going to work very slowly, touching briefly into the activating events, then backing out and doing a resourcing exercise.

Think about the moment just before impact. Now immediately think of someone who is a source of comfort and strength to you. How would it feel if they were there with you? What happens in your body when you think of them? Do you feel a loosening, a relaxing? If you do not experience a relaxation response, continue to work through your list of resources until you do.

Once you experience the relaxation response, think of the impact again. What other resources would your body want to have with you? What would make you feel safe?

If you are working with a partner, freeze-frame the first moment of impact. Have your partner help you find a resource, then ask you "What happens next?" Your partner should repeat what you have just said in the last segment: "And then you see the other car run the red light and come toward you . . . and what happens next?"

Repeat this exercise several times touching the edge of the activating event and then switching to a resource that brings relaxation. Then stop working on the accident and do another activity. Because of the amount of trapped energy, this work is very tiring. Plan to repeat the exercise for several days. When you can begin to think about the impact without feeling your body tense, your stomach churn, your breathing quicken, or other familiar symptoms, you will know that you have successfully dissipated much of the trapped energy.

Key Points

- Impact is usually the most difficult aspect of the accident to work through

- It is important to move back and forth, or loop, between experiences that are traumatic and those that are soothing

- It is common to feel fear or anger when working through the freeze response that results from impact

- Initiating and completing the preparatory or organizing movements related to the fight-or-flight responses facilitates deep discharge

12

$\backsim$

Whiplash and Compression

You may list whiplash among your accident symptoms. It's the most common complaint of auto accident victims and difficult to avoid.

At the moment of impact, you sometimes receive many physical traumas simultaneously. Whiplash is almost inevitable. Even slow-speed accidents can cause whiplash. Women are more subject to whiplash than men because they generally have longer, more slender necks and less muscle strength in the neck and upper shoulders.

What Your Neck Goes Through

Depending on the direction of the impact, your neck may have been forced rapidly backward by the force of the collision, then rapidly forward or from side to side, hyperextending the muscles and nerves in both directions. To complicate the situation, you may have been turning at the time of the accident to see the oncoming car, looking in the rear-view mirror, or forced into an awkward position by your seatbelt, creating a complicated twisting rather than a simple whiplash. You may have hit your head on the headrest or steering wheel, compounding the injuries.

When whiplash and subsequent muscular hyperextension occurs, muscles tend to constrict in an attempt to bring the weight and position of the head back to center. With whiplash, you are dealing with a mixture of overextended and overcontracted muscles.

Your neck muscles are weakened by the trauma. After experiencing whiplash, many clients describe feeling like their head is a bowling ball resting on toothpicks. Until the nervous system activation is released, other therapies such as craniosacral, chiropractic, or massage aren't as effective and may cause a reverse reaction, such as I had after my accident.

During my accident, because I was leaning over, I was twisted to the right at the moment of impact. My neck was so sore afterwards that I had a massage therapist work just on that area. After the session, I felt great! However, as I was driving home, my muscles went limp. I couldn't hold my head up at all. I literally had to hold my neck up with my hand. Later, the muscles all constricted and the pain was worse than before. The physical release felt wonderful, but my system wasn't ready for that much release and constricted again. That is why we take things one step at a time.

Brace, Collapse, and Rebound

Do you feel as if your back and neck are wooden or immobile? We often see this in our clients. They arrive in the office with neck, head, and shoulders braced. To be "braced" means to stay stiff, tense, and rigid. To see left or right, they move only their eyes or their entire bodies, not their necks. In this state, flexibility is very limited.

When you are braced, your peripheral vision is limited. This compromises your safety, especially while driving. Bracing yourself in your body is a normal reaction to threat. We have the expression "scared stiff." If trauma isn't too great the body will go through a normal sequence of bracing, then collapsing with exhaustion. It takes a lot of energy to remain braced. If a person can allow the experience of feeling collapsed, they can rebound to their normal state. Both the bracing and collapse response are normally time limited, but with trauma a person can get stuck in either or both of these states.

Try to become aware of any braced or collapsed areas in your body. Then engage the support of resources, such as the presence of a protective ally or a safe place, giving yourself time to complete the response. In this way you will move on through the sequence to the rebound response, which is defined as a return to resiliency, strength, and well-being.

Work with a partner, if possible, in the following exercise. When your body releases the bracing, you are likely to experience the collapse response. All your muscles go limp, just as mine did after the neck massage. You may feel very weak.

Let this response happen. Don't let it alarm you. It is a natural result of the release of energy, not a symptom of weakness. After a few minutes, your body should begin to feel relief, and you will experience a rebound response and feel resilient and aware of your surroundings with relaxed alertness.

Our culture tends to reward stoicism. We expect people to "just get over it." Your learned responses may make you want to brace yourself and fight against this collapse response. Experiment with giving in and letting it happen.

Exercise: Whiplash Unwound

This exercise helps unwind the whiplash. For better results use a high-backed chair that supports your head and neck. An executive-style office chair is ideal. You'll also need a pillow to support your neck because your muscles may be weak. I use a special long tube-shaped bolster that wraps around the neck and goes under the arms. A foam swimming support would be effective, or a dog-bone shaped headrest pillow. Longer pillows give you the feeling that your neck is contained.

Have your partner gently support your head in her hands. She should not attempt to move your head—your body will do this on its own during the exercise. She should, however, prevent you from moving too quickly or too far. Your neck has been hyperextended and you do not want to repeat the experience.

Remember the moment of impact. Where is your head? What is it doing? As your body remembers the accident, you will feel your head begin to move. You may feel as if your head and neck are moving your body.

> Caution: Do this exercise slowly! Do not push through pain. Stop and allow discharge if you feel pain or tension. Move back into a position where your neck can relax. Some people feel the impulse to throw their heads back as in the original whiplash. DO NOT DO THIS! Be gentle. Go slowly.

Find your most comfortable position, and then gradually expand your range of movement, as your body is ready. Re-enact the accident in slow motion. As you tap into the accident, you will feel your head want to move in an unwinding motion. Allow it to move only a little, then back out and tap into a resource until you experience a relaxation response. Repeat.

Before you end this exercise, do some of the grounding exercises from Chapter 4, feeling the sensations of your seat and feet touching the chair and floor. This helps reintegrate your upper and lower body.

David Rippe

Remember David, whose car was struck by a pick-up truck as he crossed the highway from his driveway? His vehicle was struck on the driver's side. The seat back broke away during the impact. David was gripping the steering wheel so hard that it bent. Somehow—he still isn't sure how— he suffered a concussion on the back of his head. We suspect his head may have struck the headrest just as the back of the seat broke away.

When he came for treatment, he was experiencing migraines, neck pain, and upper back spasms. His back muscles were hyperextended and constricted from having to support his body after the seat back broke off. Any movement that tipped him backward was very threatening.

I put David in a chair that tilts back. I had him relax in the chair, supported him, and tipped him back until he began to touch into whiplash activation. Using the looping technique, I then gently pushed the chair forward to allow him to relax again. After giving him plenty of time to experience the relief of discharge, I tilted him back again until he began to experience the edge of the activation. We repeated the experience, going back a bit farther each time. His back spasms were eventually greatly reduced.

After the third time I tilted David back, he began to get pain in his head, which indicated that although we had released the energy causing the back spasms, a new level of symptoms had surfaced. Symptoms that were resolved earlier may reappear during re-enactments. Stop or slow down when they do. Work on one thing at a time. Any time you do re-enactments of your accident, you are likely to experience activation and may be tired afterwards.

Often, several sessions are sufficient to relieve whiplash and back or neck spasms. In David's case, his symptoms were greatly reduced with the first treatment. He had been in chronic pain from the accident for three years before he came to therapy, so our goals were to reduce his level of pain and to extend the periods of time during which he was pain free.

Photo of David's Accident

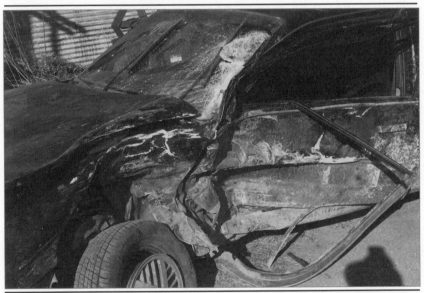

Exercise: Whiplash Release

This exercise relieves the weight of your head on your neck. It may increase your range of motion if your neck feels stuck.

Imagine your head is floating on the top of your neck. Make tiny movements forward and back, and side to side. Feel how your head seems to glide slowly and gently on fluid. Allow your head to float and your neck to support it easily. How does this feel?

Key Points

- Whiplash is a common occurrence in auto accidents and much more complicated than you may realize

- Nervous system activation plays a critical and often unrecognized role in adding to the pain of damaged muscles, tendons, and ligaments

- Other excellent approaches such as chiropractic, craniosacral therapy, physical therapy, and massage can be much more effective when nervous system overactivation is corrected

- Many auto accident survivors suffer from feeling either braced and rigid or weak and collapsed

- Normally the brace response and the collapse response are time-limited. Healing involves allowing the body time to complete this sequence and rebound to its normal state

13

⌒

Seatbelt and Airbag Injuries

Seatbelts and airbags provide increased safety and reduce the risk of injury. Sometimes they increase your trauma by making you feel trapped or and even sometimes by inflicting injury. Think about your accident for a moment. Remember the feeling of the seatbelt around you? Do you remember it feeling protective or restrictive?

Do turtlenecks or tight collars make you feel trapped since your accident? Do you get a feeling of panic every time you buckle your seatbelt? Some accident survivors report these sensations.

During an accident, your body is thrown forward, but restrained by the seatbelt in an asymmetrical position. The higher the speed of the impact, the more pressure the seatbelt exerts on your neck, chest, and abdomen. Afterward, your nervous system retains the memory of this strong pressure across your body, causing puzzling symptoms. The symptoms may be centered on the left side of your neck, or you may find your left shoulder is locked in a forward position and has chronic pain.

Once you have released the nervous system activation, chiropractic, physical therapy, or massage treatments may be helpful in relieving any remaining pain from the twisting impact.

Nancy

A year after her accident, Nancy developed stomach pains and chronically inflamed intestines. Wearing her seatbelt intensified the symptoms. Tests ruled out any medical cause for her discomfort. The accident haunted her, and she was unable to perform everyday tasks.

During treatment, I realized that Nancy had a split focus during her accident. Her young daughter, Sarah, was in the back seat, and though she knew she was unharmed, she continued to fear for Sarah's welfare. Through resourcing and visualization, seeing her daughter well, Nancy was able to resolve this conflict and fully realize that Sarah was safe, allowing her to focus more fully on her own recovery.

We then began to work on Nancy's stomach pains, using techniques of visualization and "what if" scenarios while asking "what does your body feel now?" I realized that the seatbelt pressure across her abdomen had triggered her nervous system to recall the pain of her caesarean surgery from five years prior. I asked Nancy to go back to the day of her caesarean and imagine being in control of the situation through visualizing herself in charge of the surgery. Subsequent work helped Nancy put the pain from the caesarean, as well as the accident, into the past where it belonged. Her stomach pain and intestinal inflammation disappeared.

Exercise: Seatbelt Trauma

This exercise will help you to resolve some of your symptoms by understanding how you reacted to your seatbelt at the time of your accident.

Remember the day of your accident. At the moment of impact, how does your seatbelt feel on your body? Do you feel trapped? What does your body want to happen? Visualize pushing the seatbelt away from you. What happens in your body when the belt is no longer binding you? What if someone else helps push the belt away? How does that feel?

If your shoulder and neck feel tense and cramped, try to think of an activity that is enjoyable that uses head and neck motion. Use that activity as a resource. For instance, one of my clients experienced tremendous relief in her shoulders when she visualized the way she used her shoulders, neck, and arms during snow skiing. Do you have intestinal or chest pains? Could these be linked to earlier illnesses or surgeries? What happens if you imagine yourself in control of these earlier events?

Airbags

Have you ever seen an airbag go off? Do you have any idea what it looks like, sounds like, or smells like? Most people don't. As drivers, we often find out for the first time how an airbag works at one of the most terrifying times in our life—at the moment of impact during an auto accident. Most often they save lives.

To my knowledge, few therapists have recognized the trauma caused by airbag deployment. I strongly believe that car dealerships and motor vehicle departments should conduct demo airbag operations so people know what to expect. It could be a highly effective preventative measure to alleviate unnecessary trauma.

The actual deployment is extremely dramatic. The airbag explodes out of the steering wheel or passenger dashboard, releasing a powder that looks like smoke and a chemical smell that makes some people believe their car is on fire. The airbag obscures your vision and can actually cause broken arms or bruises. Airbags have caused several deaths. Children and small or elderly drivers are at particular risk.

Adrienne

Adrienne was driving on a city street when another car coming toward her made an abrupt turn, striking her broadside. The totally unexpected impact spun her car around and forced it across the street and into the parking lot of a service station.

At the moment of impact, her airbag deployed, breaking her arm. She couldn't see over the airbag. She heard a loud explosion. Her car filled with what she thought was smoke. There was a strong chemical odor that Adrienne identified as fire. Her door was jammed. Panicked and disoriented, Adrienne flung herself across the center console in her car and out the passenger side of the car, injuring herself further. Fortunately, since the car had been pushed into a parking lot, she did not fall out into oncoming traffic. Adrienne was so terrified at the thought of her car being on fire that she didn't give a thought to what might be outside. In reality, the sound, smell, and visual obstruction that frightened her were a result of not knowing what to expect from the deployment of the airbags.

Exercise: Airbag Anxiety

This exercise helps deactivate any anxiety you may have from the deployment of your airbag.

Did your airbag deploy during your accident? Remember that instant. How does it feel? Is it protective or threatening? What happens in your body? Is there a tightening or a relaxation? What does your body want to happen? Do you want to push the airbag away? Do you want to tuck it back into the steering wheel? What do you feel when you imagine pushing the bag away? What would you want instead of the airbag? What if it had been a large feather pillow? A huge sponge? Imagine these and examine how your body feels. Does your body relax? Continue visualizing and resourcing until you do.

Key Points

- Seatbelts and airbags, though life saving, can also cause psychological trauma symptoms and physical injuries

- Sometimes unusual physical symptoms result from the abrupt pull of the seatbelt on your body

- Knowing what to expect when an airbag deploys is good preventative medicine

14

~

Road Rage

Article after article details incidents of road rage. Police launch special campaigns to catch aggressive drivers. Yet seldom do the articles address the role of trauma in road rage. I believe that a great deal of aggressive driving results from the unresolved fight-or-flight response following trauma, especially automobile accident trauma.

Some people will avoid conflict after trauma (flight response) and others will become aggressive (fight response). Until the trauma from the accident is resolved, accident victims may reenact their accident again and again.

Personality plays a role in road rage as well. People who give in to road rage are seeking an outlet for anger they haven't dealt with. It may be anger against their boss, their wife, their job, or their children. Cars give them anonymity. They are able to discharge their anger more easily with strangers.

Often this anger and rage is the consequence of feelings of helplessness and humiliation, especially for men. Instead of dealing with their feelings of inadequacy, they may try to humble or humiliate others. Backing down can seem impossible, because it would increase their own feelings of helplessness.

Susan

My friend Susan and her husband were in their car when someone cut them off in traffic. Susan's husband sped up, and cut off the other driver. They continued to cut one another off until, to her astonishment, Susan's husband reached under the seat of the car, pulled out a handgun she did not know he owned, and brandished it at the other driver. Though the gun wasn't loaded, Susan's husband was arrested for the incident.

I find that many clients also use cars as a weapon. One of my teenage clients told me that whenever he was mad, he would get into his car and drive as fast as he could, sometimes up to 120 miles an hour.

Sonja

Sonja's was a strange case. Trauma that was only incidentally related to automobiles turned into classic road rage. Sonja's marriage was in turmoil. She and her husband had separated, but animosity continued.

After an argument, Sonja was driving on the highway when her husband pulled up next to her and shot her three times. Incredibly, she was able to stop the car safely and survived her wounds. After five or six sessions she thought she was fine. During the course of our talk, she revealed that anytime she saw a car like his on the highway, she would chase it! She didn't realize that signaled a problem. She hadn't realized how her anger at her husband was causing her to act out without awareness.

Jodie

Jodie's is a classic case of trauma re-enactment. She was involved in two rear-end accidents and had not been able to resolve the anger she felt at the other drivers.

One day, Jodie was out for a drive in the mountains. She was on a dirt road miles from civilization when another car pulled up behind her and began tailgating her. Jodie got madder and madder at the other driver. Finally, she slammed on her brakes at the bottom of a hill, causing the other car to crash into hers. As a result of the accident she caused, she was in a neck brace for months—which only increased her anger.

Reworking the Anger

The main way to treat people who are prone to road rage is to help them deal with their anger in a safe environment. Often, the anger is a result of an incomplete fight-or-flight response. The pressure to complete the response builds in the nervous system, escalating rage.

Thwarted rage can become so intense that the victim can feel homicidal, with anger directed outward, or suicidal if the anger is directed internally. If you have these intense feelings of anger following an accident, you need to seek professional help and complete exercises that help you release the rage.

> NOTE: If road rage and uncontrollable anger continue to be a problem for you, you need to seek therapy if you have not already done so. Left untreated, your rage may lead you to harm yourself or others.

In the past, many therapists believed that acting out rage by pounding pillows or beating someone with foam bats was the best way to dissipate anger. In Somatic Experiencing, we believe that acting anger out explosively tends to escalate it. As pointed out earlier, it is the preparation to act, moving through the impulses slowly and with awareness, rather than the actual action of beating on something, that releases trapped energy. We do not encourage the physical acting out of anger. We offer the following exercise as an alternative.

Exercise: Fight Response

This exercise helps release trapped rage and complete the fight response.

Recall the time of your accident. When did you first begin to feel anger? Using one of the sensation exercises, change this to body sensation. What does anger feel like in your body? Do you want to hit someone? Which arm wants to hit? How?

What did you want to do to the other person in the accident? Did you want to punch them in the face? Imagine doing it. Feel your arm getting ready to move. What happens in your body?

What else might you do? One client imagined taking a machine gun and shooting out the tires of the other car, stopping the car before it hit her. Another envisioned herself running over the other car in a huge truck. Others visualize themselves as giants, capable of pushing the other car away before impact. Can you imagine doing these things? Feel your body getting ready to act. What happens in your chest? In your arms?

Continue visualizing ways to take your anger out on the other driver or car until you feel a relaxation response and a sense of strength and power. Remember, you can complete the anger related to the fight response alone or with your therapist in a safe way.

Key Points

- Road rage is often the consequence of unresolved trauma

- Working through a thwarted fight response can reduce anger and rage

- Unresolved rage from previous accidents can make you more susceptible to future accidents

15

⤴

Those Strange Symptoms

Insomnia, Weight Gain, Sexual Dysfunction, Disconnection, and Time-Space Distortions

Insomnia

Insomnia may seem like a strange reaction to an auto accident, but it is one we see often. Going to sleep involves the capacity to relax and let go. Following an accident, you may remain in a hypervigilant state, scanning constantly for danger. You can't let go, or if you do sleep, you wake abruptly with your mind going a mile a minute.

Think back to our example of how animals react to danger. If you're a gazelle and there's a cheetah nearby, you're not going to graze peacefully or lie down and sleep. You're going to be on alert for danger.

NOTE: Until excess energy is released from your nervous system following an accident, your body doesn't realize it's out of danger.

Lonnie

Lonnie was hit by a bus while crossing the street in a crosswalk. She had no warning, and was struck from behind. When she came to me, she had not slept for five straight days and couldn't understand why. She didn't believe her insomnia had anything to do with the accident. Lonnie did not realize there could be a connection between the two.

I helped her understand how her system was still in "danger mode," on full alert with her nervous system being flooded by the stimulation. We worked together until she could replay the accident with the bus at a safe distance away, giving her time to prepare for the impact—a time factor that was not present during the actual accident. Over several sessions, as she worked through her uncompleted fight-or-flight sequence, her chronic hypervigilance dissolved and her capacity to sleep was restored.

Feeling Safe Again

Like the dog we told you about in a previous chapter, we need a safe place to rest after an accident until we can discharge energy. We use a series of exercises with our clients until they can turn down their dimmer dial on their excess energy and begin to relax. (Telling a trauma victim to "Just relax" heads our list of *101 Things You Don't Say To An Accident Survivor.* Obviously if you could relax you would!)

Often, our clients become sleepy during the course of the session. They're embarrassed and apologize—but they are exhibiting the response we're working toward—the capacity to let down and rest.

Exercise: Relaxation

These exercises will help you discharge excess nervous system energy and eventually turn off your hypervigilance.

Think of creative ways you can discharge and neutralize. Try using a hot tub, getting a massage, or taking a hot bath surrounded by scented candles. (You can imagine doing these things, or actually do them, whichever is most comfortable for you.) Be sure to observe the sensations you feel in your body.

Everyone has someplace they feel especially safe. For Lonnie, this was imagining herself on a beach in Baja. Another client found she could calm herself by going to bed wrapped in comforters.

Where is your safe place? Remember a time when you felt really relaxed, slept well, and were safe. Where were you? What did it look like? What sounds could you hear? Who was with you? What happens to you when you imagine being there again?

The safest place may be one you visualize. Can you see yourself on a beach, basking in the warm sun, lying on the soft, warm sand, hearing the waves lapping gently on the shore? What happens in your body?

Imagine yourself in a mountain meadow. The cool wind whispers across your face. You smell the scent of pine. In the distance, you hear a water-fall. How does this feel in your body?

Some clients find fanciful visualizations to be calming. One woman saw herself in a four-poster bed at the side of the road, curtains blowing like in a linen ad, floating on feather comforters while she watched her accident from a distance.

Remember, when you are using resources, you can allow yourself the luxury of fantasy. You can imagine events occurring any way that brings you comfort and a relaxation response. What is important is finding any kind of image or experience that helps the nervous system discharge.

I Can't Stay Awake

You may have read the previous section in disbelief, because you not only have no trouble sleeping since your accident, but you can hardly stay awake long enough to function.

Insomnia results when your sympathetic nervous system is flooded. If your parasympathetic nervous system is overcharged, your whole system has its brakes on. You may feel heavy, lethargic, lacking energy. You often oversleep.

This signals that your system has gone into a deeply shut down state. The trapped energy is tightly bound. Some people go back and forth between the two conditions—alternating between flooding and shutdown. Your system's reaction to trauma is to narrow your world to reduce incoming stimulus. Unfortunately, the more you shut down, the less stimulation you can handle. Agoraphobia is an extreme example of this, when a person narrows their world to the extent of avoiding the world outside.

Trauma is like a tidal wave to your nervous system. You become afraid of your own bodily reactions, particularly anything that is arousing. Your anxiety about your own activation becomes the threat that overwhelms you. As Peter Levine says, "Trauma is in the body, not in the event."

When you reach this point of reaction, the smallest stimulus can be too much for your system to cope with. It is important for you to develop the capacity to allow some activation again using the exercises that we have presented to slowly discharge the arousal.

Practicing the exercises on resiliency from Chapter 7 will help you wake your system from this contracted and shutdown state.

Why Am I Gaining Weight?

Have you gained or lost weight since your accident without trying to do so? Women are especially prone to weight gain following trauma. Our bodies urge us to re-regulate the nervous system, and food is one natural form of self-medication. I gained more than 30 pounds in the months following my head-on collision. Many people choose food, drugs, or alcohol to try and lift depression.

In fact, your choice of self-medications may give you a clue to where in the nervous system your trapped energy lies. If it is in the sympathetic nervous system, making you feel "wired" or hypervigilant, you are likely to turn to "comfort foods" that contain high levels of carbohydrates and fat (i.e., pasta, bread, or ice cream). You may turn to alcohol or sleeping pills for their calming effect. On the other hand, if you are feeling shutdown or lethargic from energy trapped in the parasympathetic system, you are likely to choose high-sugar foods, caffeine, or amphetamines for their stimulating effect.

Stephen

One of my husband's clients, though not an auto accident victim, typifies the self-medication syndrome. He came to Larry for treatment of his anxiety. During discussions in their sessions, Larry learned that Stephen drank 17 cups of coffee a day and ate candy bars instead of meals. He also smoked heavily.

Once Larry understood the overt cause of Stephen's anxiety, he had him gradually cut back on caffeine. Much of Stephen's anxiety disappeared and he and Larry were able to begin work on the underlying depression that led him to feel this need for stimulation.

Why You Shouldn't Diet Now

Unfortunately, self-medications are only temporary fixes. Nevertheless, because they are your body's way to compensate and comfort, we don't recommend that you stop any of these temporary self-treatments until you've released the trapped energy from your accident. If you do, you are likely to feel out of control. This is not a time to try to impose self-discipline. You have to be ready and to feel empowered again before you can successfully overcome unhealthy habits.

Once you have resolved the trauma, you will find the need for the self-medication is gradually reduced. Most of my clients drop the weight they gained relatively easily as treatment progresses.

Why Don't I Care About Sex Anymore?

Just like sleeping, good sex requires relaxing and letting go. But unlike sleep, sex involves stimulation and arousal. Even though you may have enjoyed sex in the past, right now your body may reject any excess stimulation. Additional arousal can overwhelm your nervous system.

Sex is an outlet for normal adults to regulate their nervous systems. Climax discharges energy, and you usually feel relaxed and comfortable after sex. All of these responses are controlled by the reptilian brain that now is disrupted by trauma. It's no wonder your sex drive and responses are changed.

As with sleeping and eating, you may find that your sex drive has gone into overdrive instead of into hibernation. This may be your body's way of reaffirming that it is alive and can feel. Many people find that sex or any vigorous exercise helps discharge excess energy.

Neither extreme is normal. Until you have completed enough

resourcing exercises to discharge energy and regain balance in your nervous system, you can not expect functions controlled by the reptilian brain to work correctly again.

Communication Is Key

If it has been several months since your accident, your partner may be losing patience with your lack of interest in sex. Let your partner read this chapter. It's important for the two of you to communicate at this time. By working together, you will be able to heal the trauma to your system and regain normal sexual interest.

Exercise: Healing Sexually

This exercise will help you and your partner work gradually into healing.

Communicate with your partner about what feels soothing, safe, and calming. At this time, any physical contact may be too much for you. If so, return to Chapter 10 on boundary repair and work through those exercises. Let your partner know what is happening and that areas of your body feel threatened by physical contact.

At first, start with just holding, caressing each other, or massage. Go at your own pace and listen to your body. Attunement to your own pace and rhythm is essential. Gain your partner's cooperation and agreement not to rush. We want to avoid retraumatization.

I'm So Disoriented

Since your accident, do you feel like you never have enough time? Do you find yourself missing appointments? Are you always feeling rushed and pressured? You may be experiencing disorientation in time.

Disorientation in space is possible too. Do you feel "off" physically? Prior to the accident, were you well-coordinated and athletic, but ever since you seem to be walking into things or dropping things? Some of our clients say that they feel physically off center, almost as if they were sitting in the passenger seat while trying to drive the car.

Another experience that some people have after an auto accident falls under the category of dissociation. Many describe their vision as being blurry or fuzzy. Quite commonly the cold people feel, either all over or in particular parts of the body, reflects the shock experienced in partial dissociation. One body part may feel particularly cold or disconnected.

Others have reported feeling like they are disconnected from their entire bodies. When this is the case, it is difficult for a person at first to feel or reach their internal sensations. When we ask them what they feel in their body, their answer is "I don't know," or "I can't tell." They may say that they feel "spacey" or "zoned out."

If you feel that has been your experience as you try to do the exercises in the book, don't worry. It just means you are still in an intense part of the shock. Instead of tracking sensation in your body, you might ask yourself "what do I notice in my experience?" Keep working with your experience in the same way we have described working in the body. Slowly you will come out of shock and you will be more easily able to connect with your bodily sensations.

The only time I don't ask clients to feel their symptoms in their body is when they are in a dissociated state. You actually resource from "out there"—wherever you feel like you are stranded. In these cases, I ask, "In your experience, what do you see? What do you feel?" By working through the exercises in this manner and discharging the excess energy slowly, eventually you will feel as if you are back in your body again.

Lonnie

Lonnie, the pedestrian who was struck by a bus, reported feeling like a character in a cartoon, where the character's essence is knocked out of the body then snatched back in again. She actually recalled looking down at herself for a moment before she came back to her body.

Key Points

• Autonomic nervous system functions such as sleeping, eating, and sexuality are strongly affected by auto accidents

- Food, alcohol and drugs can be used in a misguided attempt to get the nervous system back into balance and ultimately make things worse

- Disorientation in time and space can stem from auto accident trauma

- Many auto accident survivors end up dissociated and disconnected from their bodies

- These dissociated states are a signal of extreme activation and must be worked with slowly and carefully

16

~~

Teenage Drivers

A Chapter for Parents and Their Children

Scary Statistics

Traffic accidents are a leading cause of death for persons 15 to 20 years old, according to the National Highway Traffic Safety Administration (NHTSA). That agency estimates the accident fatality rate for teen drivers (16 to 19) is almost four times that of drivers 25 through 69. Young drivers between 15 and 20 years old accounted for 6.7 percent of licensed drivers in 1996, but were involved in 14 per cent of fatal crashes, and 17 percent of all police-reported crashes. The estimated economic cost of police-reported crashes involving drivers between 15 and 20 years old was $31.9 billion in 1997, per NHTSA figures.

Furthermore, almost one-third of the 15- to 20-year-old drivers involved in fatal crashes had an invalid license at the time of the crash. Almost 30 percent of those in the 15 to 20 age group who were killed in motor vehicle crashes had been drinking.

Expert Advice

Because teenage drivers have such high accident and fatality rates, we consulted a colleague with special expertise in this area, Jim Jonell, Ph.D., a specialist in adolescent psychotherapy.

According to Dr. Jonell, a major cause of teenage accidents is the assumption on the part of parents, insurance companies, and the legislature that all children are ready to get behind the wheel of a car at age 16. In fact, Dr. Jonell points out, many teens do not have the emotional maturity at this age to be handed a lethal weapon and pointed toward the roads. Further, many mid-teens lack the physical reflexes to react quickly in driving situations. Yet most parents can't imagine saying no to their children who want driver's licenses as soon as they are eligible. "Some parents won't even let a kid stay home alone, but will turn them loose with a car," Dr. Jonell said.

Dr. Jonell's own son was the only one of six friends who didn't have a major accident within the first six months of getting his license. The others seemed to feel accidents were a normal part of teen driving. The consequences most of these children faced following their accidents were minimal. Most were given new cars.

Dr. Jonell further advises that licenses be denied to children who have proven a lack of responsibility, especially those who have criminal records. Read the accident statistics at the beginning of this chapter again, and note the number of teens with suspended or invalid licenses and those where alcohol was involved.

What Parents Can Do

Dr. Jonell offers several tips for parents to help their teens become safer drivers:

- Model good driving behavior. Do you wear your seatbelt? Do you tailgate or make obscene gestures? Do you cut into traffic or swear at other drivers? Do your children see you doing this?

- Maintain control of the car keys. The Jonell children did not get their own cars until they were 21. Whenever Dr. Jonell had an issue with his children, he took the car keys off the peg where they usually hung. They had to come to him, ask what the problem was, and resolve the issue before keys were returned.

- Let teenagers deal with the consequences of their behavior. Don't rescue them whenever they get a ticket.

- Make rules for behavior in the car, and insist that teens enforce the rules when their friends are with them. Rules might include no eating, drinking, talking on the cell phone, or smoking while driving; no distracting the driver by talking to him or her; no shrieking or sudden loud noises.

- Teach your children to refuse to get into a car with any driver who has been drinking.

- Be tuned in to what is going on in your children's lives. Restrict driving during times they are under extreme stress.

- Do not laugh it off if underage children "borrow" the car while you are gone. Stealing a car is a felony. Not only is it a serious legal offense, but also a sign of immaturity and irresponsibility.

If Your Child Has an Accident

Some teenagers deal with accidents well, others do not. The difference, Dr. Jonell believes, is how their parents react. This is not the time to blame or accuse your child. He or she needs your support, and for you to remain as calm and gentle as possible. It's natural for you to be angry—it's part of the protective response parents have toward their young—but it's important for your child to get comfort from you at this time. "Ask yourself who's really important here," Dr. Jonell said. "Your child has been damaged. You have to put your own feelings aside. Find someone else to give you support—you must be supportive to your child. Don't retraumatize them with your reaction. Create a healing environment."

Fathers may have a harder time dealing with their anger. Dr. Jonell recalls one of his clients who was injured in an accident, and was in a coma.

Dr. Jonell and the boy's father met in the hospital room, where the father gave in to his anger, blaming his son for the accident. Dr. Jonell insisted they leave the room.

"But he's in a coma. He can't hear me," the father said.
"Yes, he can," Dr. Jonell replied, leading him from the room.

After venting his anger, the father went back into the room, hugged his son, and began to sob. Just then, the boy regained consciousness.

Be alert for symptoms of trauma months after the accident, Jonell cautions. Though your child may insist everything is fine, his or her system has suffered a severe stress. Grades and athletic activities may not reflect the trauma, but it may manifest itself in loss of appetite, sleep difficulties, or changes in relationships with family and friends.

Dr. Jonell remembers the first time his daughter stayed out past her midnight curfew. By 3 a.m., he was terrified, imagining all sorts of horrible scenarios. When she got home, he first felt frozen, then anger, then fear. Finally, he threw his arms around her, hugged her, and started to cry. She was stunned by his reaction, explained that she had fallen asleep on the couch at her boyfriend's house, and they proceeded to discuss the situation calmly.

Jim

Jim Jonell knows from personal experience that symptoms of auto accident trauma can surface many years after the accident. When Jim was 14, he was in an accident on the way back home from a church trip. He was asleep in the back seat and a youth leader was driving. Truck lights blinded the driver at an intersection and the car spun out of control, hitting a light pole and knocking electrical wires down into the highway.

The passenger in the front seat was thrown through the windshield and killed. Jim, wakened from sleep by the accident, was unharmed and able to run to a nearby house for help. By the time he returned to the scene, firemen and police had arrived. Jim got there in time to see a state trooper reach for the car door and die by electrocution. To this day, Jim has no idea how he got out of the car without being electrocuted.

Jim says his follow-up care was excellent. He got medical care for his minor injuries and counseling for the trauma. He thought he was fine, until at age 29, he fell asleep in the back seat of a car. His wife stepped on the brakes, jolting him awake. He woke screaming, though there was no danger or impact. Jim realized that he was having a flashback to his accident and needed more work before the incident was resolved in his nervous system.

Damien

When Damien came to Dr. Jonell for treatment, he didn't think his accident bothered him at all. In fact, he thought the whole thing was rather amusing, like playing bumper cars. However, since the accident he had developed a severe stutter.

Dr. Jonell asked Damien to tell him about the accident. As he did, the muscles in his jaw tightened and his stuttering became more pronounced. As they discussed the accident, Damien realized that he had wanted to go home, tell his mother about the accident, and have her make everything okay. Instead, she reacted with anger, which made all his muscles tighten and caused the stutter.

Often, an accident survivor thinks he or she has no residual difficulties from the accident, but seemingly unimportant little physical quirks may prove otherwise.

Tonya

One of our clients, Tonya, was involved in a serious auto accident in her teens. She was thrown through the windshield and had to undergo a series of plastic surgeries to repair her face. When she started treatment, though she thought she had no lasting problems from the accident, we noticed that at each session she was clutching a small fragment of glass from the broken windshield. She rubbed this token of the event like a worry stone. Her unrecognized stress was so severe that the glass was worn smooth from her rubbing.

There's Good News

One technique that Dr. Jonell often uses with young clients is to take them driving. Their parents want him to take away all the anxiety from their accident, but his goal is to help them control their feelings. Often, the child emerges from the accident a better driver, slower and more cautious. As we discuss in the chapter on transformation, accidents can change lives in positive as well as negative ways.

Louise

Louise's auto accident was transformational. In college, Louise saw herself as plump and unattractive. She was shy and quiet. Though she had women friends, she seldom dated. Early in her sophomore year of college, Louise and a group of girlfriends went on a picnic with a group of boys from a neighboring college. Rushing to get back before curfew, the driver of the car Louise was in missed a curve and plunged into the road bank. Louise was thrown through the window, slicing her face on the glass.

The driver and his fraternity brothers virtually adopted Louise during the weeks she was hospitalized. They visited, socialized, and brought gifts. Convinced that she was hideously scarred, Louise decided that no one would ever like her for the way she looked. (After plastic surgery, her facial scar was barely visible.)

Instead of falling into despair, Louise began to exert herself to be liked in spite of her looks. Louise transformed into an outgoing young woman, popular with men and women alike. A talented singer, she performed in coffeehouses. Louise went on to marry one of the fraternity men and have a successful career in finance after graduation.

Key Points

- Young drivers are involved in a disproportionate percentage of auto accidents

- Children should not be allowed to drive until they are clearly emotionally and physically ready

- A young person who has been in an accident will often develop symptoms that a parent needs to be alert to

- If your child has been in an accident, you can use techniques in this book, such as resourcing, to help them recover

17

~

An Accident
where Someone Died

A Special Chapter

Were you in an accident where someone died? If so, there are two powerful themes that you have to deal with for your own recovery. The first is how to manage your grief. The second is how to deal with the guilt. Most people feel guilt after an accident where someone died, whether or not they were in any way to blame.

Respecting the Need to Grieve

It is not within the scope of this book to deal with the complexity of the grief process. There are many excellent books available, and if you feel yourself struggling with grief, we urge you to seek out additional resources on this subject. We simply want to highlight a few points that you may find helpful in dealing with this complex and difficult aspect of recovery.

First, in our "get over it" culture, it's important to emphasize that grieving is something we need to allow when we've experienced loss, and that sometimes the grieving process may take years.

Larry talks about the "gate effect" of grieving. Normally, right after a terrible loss, we're too numb to feel any real grief. The gates are still closed.

Over the years, many of our clients have felt that something was wrong with them because they weren't able to cry over the loss of a loved one, and had been judged harshly by others because of it. Not being able to cry often means that a person is still in deep shock.

Other people may react with anger, withdrawal, dissociation, or depression. As long as a person doesn't stay stuck in these states for a long period of time, these states can be part of the normal healing process. It's only when people stay stuck in these states for an indefinite period that we know the grieving process is not progressing normally.

Real grieving doesn't usually begin until several months after loss. The gates will begin to open. We can only tolerate for so much grief to come through these gates at any one time, and each person is different in his or her capacity to let the grief come through. It's important to let the grief come through, not to deny it, but not to push yourself either. The gate opening and closing is a natural physiological and psychological process.

In the first year after loss, holidays, birthdays, or shared events will be among the many triggers that caused the gates to open, and that's natural and as it should be. It's better if you can just allow the grief to surface. Slowly, over time, the flood of grief will diminish, but even years later certain triggers may open the gates in a way that you may find surprising and unexpected.

I'm Glad I Survived—But Don't Tell Anyone

The second difficult aspect that seems to come up when someone died is guilt. How you deal with guilt depends on the circumstances of the accident. This guilt people feel, even if they were not at fault, is called "survivor guilt." Sometimes you might feel that you don't deserve to live if someone else has died. You may question, "Why you and not me?" Survivor guilt can result from an unconscious feeling of relief that though someone died, it wasn't you.

If a loved one or best friend died in the accident, your guilt feelings will be intense. They will be even worse if the accident was your fault. But perhaps the greatest source of most people's guilt feelings is what we call "survivor guilt," a secret feeling of relief that if someone died, it was them and not you.

Most people find this thought so repugnant, so repulsive, that they suppress it or are further traumatized by having such ideas. What is important to understand is that we're internally dedicated to self-preservation. Our entire biology is programmed to take the actions necessary to keep us alive during traumatic events. Afterward it's natural for us to be glad that we survived.

Though the "I'm glad I survived" thought is biologically induced, we feel ashamed of ourselves for thinking it when someone in the accident died. It's natural to be glad. Surviving feels good. It does not mean that we're glad something bad happened to someone else.

Before we can move on, it's important to realize that we don't have control over life and death. It's a degree of helplessness we have to accept. Sometimes an accident is our fault—as mine was. Fortunately for both of us, the other driver lived.

You need to understand that this "thank God it wasn't me" feeling arises from your self-preservation instinct. It's a natural response. On the very deepest level, our drive to survive is so powerful that we can't help but rejoice that we are alive. It's a manifestation of our will to live. For our biological and animal selves, survival is success.

Acknowledge to yourself that you are thankful to be alive. Your pleasure in surviving does not mean that you are happy someone else died. Don't blame yourself if someone died; you did not want to harm anyone. You need to grieve the tragedy.

Harriet

Harriet was in a sports car driven by her boyfriend, David, in the mountains of New Mexico. Neither was wearing a seatbelt. The road was steep and winding. David swerved to avoid a deer in the road and the car went into a ditch. Both Harriet and David were ejected from the car. David was killed in the accident, while Harriet, although seriously injured, survived. Gradually, she realized that her survival did not mean "David's death."

Harriet continued to have strange aches and pains a year and a half after the accident. She thought they were a result of her injuries, but medical doctors pronounced her free of physical problems. She went to many doctors seeking relief before she entered therapy with Larry.

As they began to explore her feelings about the accident, it became clear that the hardest thing for Harriet to acknowledge was that she was glad she survived. She realized that she wished that she, not David, had been killed. When she came close to admitting that she was glad she was alive, her symptoms became worse.

Harriet and Larry worked through the accident piece by piece, stopping to use her resources frequently until she could recount the events without becoming agitated. After several sessions, Harriet was able to recognize that she did indeed rejoice in her own survival though she still mourned David's death. Eventually her symptoms were alleviated.

Guilt by Observation

You don't have to be involved in an accident to feel survivor guilt. Simply witnessing it can be enough.

Greg

Greg and his sister were playing near their home when his sister darted out into the street. She was struck by a truck and killed. Greg's grief and guilt were so severe that he developed chronic migraines. Through therapy, he came to terms with his survivor guilt and was able to acknowledge that he was glad he was alive. His migraines disappeared, though milder headaches did return when he was under stress.

NOTE: Symptoms may return at a later time, though usually much less severe. The return of symptoms may signal a need to do more work to release trapped energy in your nervous system.

Guilt Comes in Many Forms

Not all post-accident guilt is survivor guilt from the death of someone close. The death of a stranger can be equally devastating. One of my patients, Patty, came to me following her accident. We found that the recent accident triggered symptoms from a car crash she had as a teenager.

Patty

Sixteen-year-old Patty had just gotten her license. She was driving out in the country on a narrow, winding road when a wide motor home came toward her, forcing her off onto the shoulder of the road. Patty overcorrected when steering back onto the highway, veering into the oncoming traffic lane momentarily.

Unfortunately, at that moment a motorcyclist came around the blind curve. Patty's car struck and killed him. Everyone in her small town knew about the accident, but no one would talk to Patty about it. Apparently they were trying to protect her feelings because they felt the accident was unavoidable. She felt isolated, alone, and guilt-ridden.

The accident changed the course of Patty's life. She changed her career decisions, feeling she had to lead the young victim's life for him since it was her fault he had died.

Patty didn't realize how much the accident affected her until, at age 38, she was involved in another traffic accident. During our treatment sessions, her memories of the earlier accident surfaced. We needed to deal with both events before she could fully recover.

One of Patty's main problems was that she felt she deserved to be in the second accident. She had been expecting it for years. Every time her husband or son left the house to drive somewhere, she feared for their safety. Patty felt so guilty about causing someone's death that she believed she deserved to be punished.

Dealing with Others in the Car

One of the complexities of auto accidents is that your anxieties may be fixated on someone else who was in the car, like passengers, children, or pets.

Elena

In her rear-view mirror, Elena saw a car behind her careening out of control. It swerved from one lane to the next. She thought it would miss her, but just as it reached her car, it swung into her path, sending Elena's car into a spin. Her young daughter, Roberta, was in the back seat. She was uninjured and seemed to consider the whole accident a great adventure akin to a carnival ride.

Elena, who was hurt in the crash, was so scared about Roberta that she couldn't deal with her own physical reactions. Though she knew on a conscious level that her daughter was fine, each time we began to work on the accident, her first question was, "Is Roberta okay?"

When we are really "freaked out" by events, our bodies get stuck in or before the trauma. Part of you actually gets frozen in time when you get overwhelmed by trauma. You may have blanked out events, so your body never gets to the end of the story. There are gaps in your experience. That is why you may not be able to move forward in time, unable to realize on a biological level that others in the car are safe and that you also survived. Elena's fear for her daughter during the accident made it impossible for her to come to completion over the events.

Anger and Blame

When anger and blame are not worked through as part of a person's recovery, there can be devastating consequences. Two of our patients experienced this in different ways.

Molly

Molly and her husband, Fred, were returning from visiting friends late at night, their car filled with potted plants they had been given. Molly asked her husband if he was too tired to drive, but he assured her that he was fine. Molly removed her seatbelt, tilted the seat back, and went to sleep.

She woke as the car was flipping through the air, landing upside down. Fred had fallen asleep and veered into the oncoming lane, then swerved back, landing in the median. Molly was totally disoriented. It was dark and objects were flying around the car. Dirt from the plants got into her eyes and she couldn't see.

Molly suffered a brain injury. She had to give up her teaching career. She was furious with her husband. She felt betrayed and never was able to resolve her anger, which seriously threatened their marriage.

Karen

Karen dropped her children off at the elementary school the morning of her accident. As she pulled out into traffic, another car veered into her lane.

A teenage boy drove the oncoming car. His sister, riding in the passenger seat, had dropped a cigarette on the floor and both of them were scrambling for it when the car went out of control.

The sister was killed in the accident. Though the teenage boy was at fault, his mother blamed Karen for his sister's death. Karen was knocked unconscious in the accident. When she awoke in the hospital she could not remember if her children had been in the car with her or not.

When she began treatment, we had to deal with Karen's tremendous guilt and her fears for her children's safety before we could relieve her accident symptoms.

What to Do about Guilt

Dealing with your guilt from an accident where someone died is one of the most difficult things you will have to face. Your reptilian brain may be telling you "I'm glad I survived," but your conscious mind rejects this thought as embarrassing, and sometimes interprets it as "I deserve to have something bad happen to me."

Guilt often results from feelings of rage and helplessness. Our anger at God or the universe for allowing something so terrible to happen often gets turned back on ourselves because we don't want to feel angry at God, or we might even be scared to feel that kind of anger.

We also often have difficulty coming to terms with the helplessness we feel when something terrible happens. Rather than acknowledge the helplessness, we may feel guilty. Guilt feels bad but it maintains the illusion of control. We weren't *really* helpless, we just did the wrong thing, we think. This belief can be particularly difficult when in hindsight we see options that we didn't perceive at the time of the accident.

Letting go of guilt means acknowledging our anger, even at God. It means accepting human fallibility, particularly our own. It means seeing that accidents are unintentional. Accidents are awful things that happen. It is important to try to come to peace with the consequences, even though that is not always an easy process.

Key Points

- When someone dies in an accident there are special considerations, such as grief and guilt, that need to be handled for complete recovery

- "Survivor guilt" involves our deep desire to survive

- Blame and anger need to be resolved for complete recovery. It is often unconscious and presents a hidden challenge for many auto accident survivors

- Guilt is often the result of rage and helplessness that we haven't been able to acknowledge and deal with

18

Achieving Transformation

When you started reading this book, you probably were anxious and frightened by the strange symptoms you were feeling. Perhaps you were stressed or having difficulty functioning in everyday activities.

By this time, you know that your symptoms and anxieties are normal physiological reactions to trauma. For many people, just knowing that they are not going crazy helps reduce symptoms.

We hope that the exercises you have been doing as you read each chapter have discharged the energy trapped in your nervous system and brought you back into balance. While some physical injuries may still hamper your activities, continued practice of the resourcing exercises should reduce symptoms arising from nervous system overload. When you can think or talk about your accident without experiencing anxiety, rapid breathing, or stomach pains, and when you feel as if the accident is in the past, you will know that you have succeeded. Better yet, the energy you were devoting to symptoms is now available to use for positive activities.

Our greatest hope for you, though, is that this book will have led you to experience transformation such as that experienced by many of Larry's and my clients. They report that healing from their accident leaves their lives changed in a positive way. I know that when you first began to read this book, it was impossible for you to envision a time when your accident might be a positive experience for you. Here's what happened to some of the people we worked with.

Lorraine

Lorraine was one of those people who always seemed driven. She was in constant motion. She could never do enough or do it right enough. She was judgmental of herself and almost totally disconnected from her body. She resented having to listen to her body's signals. Lorraine felt she was the master and her body her slave. If she was tired, she simply worked harder and longer. She felt tireless because she refused to listen to her body's signs of exhaustion. It's a lifestyle that is rewarded in our society, one that views pushing through pain as admirable.

After her accident, Lorraine resented her body even more. She felt betrayed by her physical weakness. But due to her injuries and symptoms, Lorraine had no choice. She had to listen to her body's needs.

Gradually, as we worked with her resources, Lorraine began to see her body as an ally rather than a slave. She began to see that her body had a wisdom she never realized was there. Her relationship with her body changed radically. She began to rest when she was tired, eat when she was hungry. Listening to her body brought balance to her life and great relief.

Lorraine had been irritable and grouchy before the accident. Afterward, she became a much happier person. She was more patient with her husband, children, and the patients in her nursing work. Most amazing of all, she came to see the accident as a gift.

"If it hadn't been for the accident, I never would have discovered myself," Lorraine told me.

Lee Daniels

Lee wanted us to use her real name to tell the story of her accident and transformative recovery.

Lee was riding her bike when she was struck by a car going 42 miles an hour. She landed on the hood of the car and smashed into the wind-

shield with her head. Then she flipped over the top of the car, landing on the pavement. Lee suffered a serious brain injury. She was also going through a divorce at the time, so the events preceding her accident also were traumatic.

Always a religious person, Lee found that her accident deepened her faith. She reports feeling the presence of a protective force throughout the accident.

Not only did a police car pass by at the time of the accident, but a nurse was on the corner across the street, witnessed the incident, and gave supportive care immediately. This support provided a positive resource for her in working through the accident.

When Lee first came to me, she was very fragmented. She spoke in bursts, like a popcorn popper. It was difficult at first to follow her story. After the early work we did, she was able to describe her experience coherently. Her outlook now is positive and enthusiastic. As a result of the accident, she is a much more confident person, bolstered by the feeling that she is cared for and protected. She knows that she has dealt with one of the most difficult things that a person has to face in this life, that she has come through it, and that she has done more than just survive.

"These two experiences of the divorce and the bike accident have permanently altered my life," she says. "I have grown, learned, forgiven, and come out knowing I was meant to have these experiences for my 'soul growth.'" "I'm emotionally stronger than I've ever been in my life. I'm very happy to be alive to experience all the exciting people, joy, and the freedom to be me!"

David Rippe

David Rippe, whose story you have read in previous chapters, says that now he has a feeling of having a way out, a feeling of being alive, and a sense of "What's next?" His life now revolves around aliveness, not pain. That sense of expectation and planning a future is diagnostic of completing the process of recovery. The accident still is scary, but no longer a huge obstacle for him. He feels like it's in the past. The trauma no longer is in the forefront of his life.

Before treatment, David felt stuck in anger. He was trapped in a fear-

aggressive state. Now it is much easier for him to maintain a state of calmness and patience. He actually feels the healing that has happened.

Learning that People Care

Sometimes an accident brings out the best in those around you. Many clients report being helped by witnesses who went out of their way to assist. One woman who was in an accident several blocks from home was unable to reach her husband by cell phone, so a witness ran to the house to get him.

We have been told many stories of good Samaritans who rendered instant help to our clients, from truckers prying out one client from a burning car to doctors, nurses, and EMTs stopping to lend a helping hand.

We've become so autonomous as a society that we sometimes don't like people helping us—and we don't like needing help or asking for it. We try to look fine and act fine, even when we are not. We don't expect to be helped, and it can be very reassuring to find that when we really do need aid that total strangers become positive resources for us.

How Does it Feel when I'm Healed?

Are you healed yet? How will you know? Go back slowly through your accident. Check for signs of activation, like anxiety, tension in any part of your body, constriction in your chest, or quickened breathing.

When you are able to stay present and resourced and the accident feels over and in the past, then you are done. You should have a feeling of "That's over and done and I'm fine now."

You should be able to drive past the location where the accident occurred without feeling symptoms. You should have no triggers that activate you, like driving, weather, or traffic.

When you have resolved your accident, you no longer will be avoiding old triggers. You can do the things you need to do and have a realistic view of risk. You should be able to eat and sleep normally and have no chronic tension. Your relationships should be back to normal, or even better than before. You should have emotional equilibrium and the resiliency to work through setbacks and pains. You should have a positive sense of self. One of the most common complaints we have heard is that after the accident, people feel that their life seems like it stopped. We hope that you are now feeling like you have your life back.

Use this resolution survey to help determine the extent of your healing. Repeat it again in several weeks.

Resolution Survey

Assess the degree to which your trauma symptoms have resolved. with this chart. "0" means you do not feel this; "5" means this strongly expresses your feelings.

	0	1	2	3	4	5
1. Sense of personal power (empowerment)	0	1	2	3	4	5
2. Able to manage challenging events	0	1	2	3	4	5
3. Realistic sense of being in control	0	1	2	3	4	5
4. Ability to focus and concentrate	0	1	2	3	4	5
5. Ability to comprehend instructions or information	0	1	2	3	4	5
6. Feeling oriented to surroundings, able to find new locations	0	1	2	3	4	5
7. Able to keep track of belongings (car keys, glasses, etc.)	0	1	2	3	4	5

8. Experience of flow or fluidity in body	0	1	2	3	4	5
9. Accurate sequential memory of events	0	1	2	3	4	5
10. Return to normal dream life	0	1	2	3	4	5
11. Absence of flashbacks	0	1	2	3	4	5
12. Uninterrupted, satisfying sleep	0	1	2	3	4	5
13. Rested, energy to function	0	1	2	3	4	5
14. Emotional equilibrium	0	1	2	3	4	5
15. Appropriate anger for situation	0	1	2	3	4	5
16. Relaxed alertness when not engaged in threat	0	1	2	3	4	5
17. Feeling safer	0	1	2	3	4	5
18. Normal startle response, lack of jumpiness	0	1	2	3	4	5
19. Feeling a sense of having choices and options	0	1	2	3	4	5
20. Feeling connected to your body	0	1	2	3	4	5
21. Feeling a sense of self	0	1	2	3	4	5
22. Sense of capability	0	1	2	3	4	5
23. Clarity and integration	0	1	2	3	4	5

24. Freedom of motion	0	1	2	3	4	5
25. Lack of recurring tension or pain patterns	0	1	2	3	4	5
26. Feeling you can orient in time	0	1	2	3	4	5
27. Feeling you can orient in space (less accident-prone)	0	1	2	3	4	5
28. Feeling connected to self	0	1	2	3	4	5
29. Feeling connected to others	0	1	2	3	4	5
30. Can discuss traumatic event without being overwhelmed	0	1	2	3	4	5
31. Traumatic event feels over	0	1	2	3	4	5
32. Able to engage more fully in normal life activities	0	1	2	3	4	5
33. Feeling calmer	0	1	2	3	4	5
34. Lack of anxiety or panic	0	1	2	3	4	5
35. Lack of unusual irritability	0	1	2	3	4	5
36. Normal eating patterns restored	0	1	2	3	4	5
37. Satisfying sexual patterns restored	0	1	2	3	4	5
38. Self-esteem versus shame	0	1	2	3	4	5
39. Ability to cope	0	1	2	3	4	5

		0	1	2	3	4	5
40.	Enjoying being with others	0	1	2	3	4	5
41.	Chronic pain alleviated, reduced, or manageable	0	1	2	3	4	5
42.	Normal level of cautiousness and vigilance	0	1	2	3	4	5
43.	Functioning support system	0	1	2	3	4	5
44.	Capacity to be present, open, and vulnerable	0	1	2	3	4	5
45.	Compassion toward self and situation	0	1	2	3	4	5
46.	Interest in life	0	1	2	3	4	5
47.	Appropriate levels of fear	0	1	2	3	4	5
48.	Appropriate levels of anger versus overreacting	0	1	2	3	4	5
49.	Intact relationships	0	1	2	3	4	5
50.	Ability to be alone comfortably	0	1	2	3	4	5
51.	Bonding with others through resiliency	0	1	2	3	4	5
52.	Feeling supportive of self and others	0	1	2	3	4	5
53.	Sense of personal future	0	1	2	3	4	5
54.	Feeling creative	0	1	2	3	4	5

55. Feeling optimistic and hopeful   0   1   2   3   4   5

56. Body feels strong
and connected   0   1   2   3   4   5

57. Capable of making decisions   0   1   2   3   4   5

58. Planning
and completing projects   0   1   2   3   4   5

59. Feeling within your personal
range of resiliency   0   1   2   3   4   5

60. Able to ask for help   0   1   2   3   4   5

61. Able to identify
and expand resources   0   1   2   3   4   5

62. Able to say no easily   0   1   2   3   4   5

63. Continuity of thought   0   1   2   3   4   5

64. Accessing appropriate
vocabulary   0   1   2   3   4   5

65. Coherent   0   1   2   3   4   5

66. Feeling present in body   0   1   2   3   4   5

67. Able to tolerate expansion   0   1   2   3   4   5

68. Able to move forward in life   0   1   2   3   4   5

69. Movement feels freer, easier   0   1   2   3   4   5

70. Ability to function at work   0   1   2   3   4   5

71. Ability to function in relationships	0	1	2	3	4	5
72. Capacity to tolerate pleasure	0	1	2	3	4	5
73. Enjoy surroundings and activities	0	1	2	3	4	5
74. Able to process stimuli comfortably	0	1	2	3	4	5
75. Comfortable in driving situations	0	1	2	3	4	5
76. Feel engaged in life	0	1	2	3	4	5
77. Able to drive by site of accident or event	0	1	2	3	4	5
78. Not afraid of the unknown	0	1	2	3	4	5
79. Willing to listen, take in calmly	0	1	2	3	4	5
80. Energy vs. chronic exhaustion	0	1	2	3	4	5
81. Able to create and access resources	0	1	2	3	4	5
82. Return readily to relaxation response after startle or threat	0	1	2	3	4	5
83. Feel curiosity, desire to explore	0	1	2	3	4	5
84. Have sense of personal space, boundaries	0	1	2	3	4	5

85. Challenges feel manageable   0   1   2   3   4   5

86. Trauma memory
    is less threatening   0   1   2   3   4   5

87. Word recall, clarity of thought   0   1   2   3   4   5

88. Shoulders and neck strengthened,
    whiplash resolved   0   1   2   3   4   5

89. Restored capacity to rest   0   1   2   3   4   5

90. Relief from addictive behaviors   0   1   2   3   4   5

91. Relief from compulsive,
    controlling behavior   0   1   2   3   4   5

92. Calmness of mind   0   1   2   3   4   5

93. Sense of empathy, compassion,
    and acceptance
    regarding suffering   0   1   2   3   4   5

94. Sense of personal
    pacing and rhythm   0   1   2   3   4   5

95. Increased patience
    and sense of ease or flow   0   1   2   3   4   5

96. Sense of closure with unsettling
    events and people   0   1   2   3   4   5

97. Connection to oneself   0   1   2   3   4   5

98. Can review traumatic incident
    without activation or distress   0   1   2   3   4   5

99. Increased confidence	0	1	2	3	4	5

100. Able to distinguish between what you can and cannot control	0	1	2	3	4	5

The higher your score, the more complete your recovery. The responses you marked 0, 1, and 2 indicate areas that you may want to continue to develop. It is often useful to retake the survey periodically to evaluate your continued progress.

Exercise: Completing Experiences

This exercise will show you the difference between completed work and incomplete experiences.

Think of some difficult experience from your past that you know is resolved—a job loss, a marital problem, an injury. How does it feel in your body when you think about this? What happens in your chest? To your breathing and heart rate? To your stomach? If the incident is mostly resolved, you should notice little or no distress.

Think of a current difficulty, something you know is not resolved. Repeat the scan of your body. What different reactions do you notice?

Use your resourcing exercises and visualization to help you resolve the current problem.

Applying Resourcing to Your Life

The resourcing exercises in this book can be used to regain resiliency in many life situations. They can guide you through times of stress and difficult choices.

Exercise: Using the Techniques

This exercise shows you how to use the techniques from this book in your daily life.

Think of any decision you have made recently. Now take it to the sensation level. How does your body feel when you think about this decision? What happens in your chest? Your heart? Your lungs? Does it feel expansive and positive?

If it does not, visualize making the opposite choice. How does this feel? Review your body's reactions.

You can use this technique to gain your body's wisdom about any choices that face you. Intuition is often a result of people being more in tune with their bodies and registering the emotional aspects that people who tend to be more mental, ignore. You can learn to deepen and strengthen this physical connection.

Envisioning the Future

Recovery means more than fixing your trauma. It's a good idea to envision the new life you want. When you are in trauma, you have no sense of the future. Part of the treatment is to think of your future. Visualize what your new life might be like.

Human beings tend to believe they are invincible. A serious accident strips that invincibility away from us. We have to recreate our boundaries and reestablish our feelings of safety. Often, an accident makes us slow down and take stock of our lives. What is working in your life? What are your priorities in life? What do you really want?

What You've Gained

When you have lived through a terrible experience and recovered from it, you have gained access to resources you never knew were there. You have learned how resilient your body is, and by listening to your body you have tapped into wisdom that will prove useful in other parts of your life. You have gained tools you didn't have before.

Trauma deepens our experience. We may come out of it with a new sense of priorities and feeling more alive than ever before. You have the confidence and knowledge that you can be deeply hurt, but recover. You have a power that those who haven't experienced trauma may never have.

Conclusion

If this book has helped you overcome your trauma, please let us know. We hope we have moved through this experience as partners, and we want to hear from you.

Visit our web site at:

www.traumasolutions.com

Diane Poole Heller, Ph.D.
Laurence Heller, Ph.D.
Rocky Mountain Psychotherapy Associates
5801 E. Ithaca Place
Denver, CO 80237

Note that the forms in this book are protected under copyright law. Please contact us if you would like additional copies of the following forms:

Trauma Symptom Survey
Client Accident Interview Form
Resolution Survey
Heller Resiliency Scan

Index

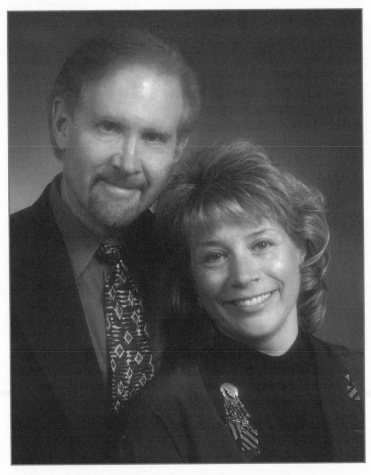

Doctors Laurence and Diane Heller

About the Authors

Dr. Diane Heller received her Ph.D. from the Western Institute for Social Research in Berkeley, California. She is a Licensed Professional Counselor and a Nationally Certified Counselor.

Heller is a faculty member and international teacher for the non-profit Foundation for Human Enrichment, founded by Peter A. Levine, Ph.D. She specializes in teaching health professionals how to work with the aftermath of trauma. She teaches regularly in Denmark, Germany, Israel, New York City, and other centers around the world.

Heller's videotape, *Columbine: Surviving the Trauma,* features her work with Columbine survivors. This video has been used as an educational tool to help the general public learn how to better cope with trauma. It was aired internationally on CNN. She has published numerous articles, manuals, and video training tapes on many aspects of healing trauma.

Dr. Laurence Heller is a Phi Beta Kappa graduate of the University of Colorado. He has an M.A. in Linguistics and a Ph.D. in Psychology. In 1972 Heller co-developed, and subsequently became the president of The Gestalt Institute of Denver. He has served as a faculty member for several American universities and teaches for the Foundation for Human Enrichment. He has trained thousands of mental health professionals over the past twenty-nine years, currently specializing in teaching therapists how to work with the aftereffects of trauma. He regularly leads trainings in the United States and throughout Europe.

Heller is fluent in Spanish and French, and teaches in these and other languages. He and his wife Diane recently taught their *Auto Accident Recovery Program* at Sarah Herzog Hospital in Jerusalem.